Losing Weight for Women:

Achieving Your Ideal Weight with Simple Home Workouts

By: Jasmin W. Alcantara

Copyright

Disclaimer

The information provided in the " Losing Weight for Women" is for general informational purposes only. While every effort has been made to ensure the accuracy and completeness of the content, the author makes no representations or warranties of any kind, express or implied, about the completeness, accuracy, reliability, suitability, or availability with respect to the information, products, services, or related graphics contained in this book for any purpose.

Any reliance you place on such information is therefore strictly at your own risk. In no event will the author be liable for any loss or damage, including without limitation, indirect or consequential loss or damage, or any loss or damage whatsoever arising from loss of data or profits arising out of, or in connection with, the use of this book.

Through this book, you may be able to link to other websites that are not under the control of the author. The author has no control over the nature, content, and availability of those sites. The inclusion of any links does not necessarily imply a recommendation or endorse the views expressed within them.

Every effort is made to keep the book up and running smoothly. However, the author takes no responsibility for, and will not be liable for, the book being temporarily unavailable due to technical issues beyond our control.

The views expressed in this book are those of the author and do not necessarily reflect the official policy or position of any other agency, organization, employer, or company.

About the Author

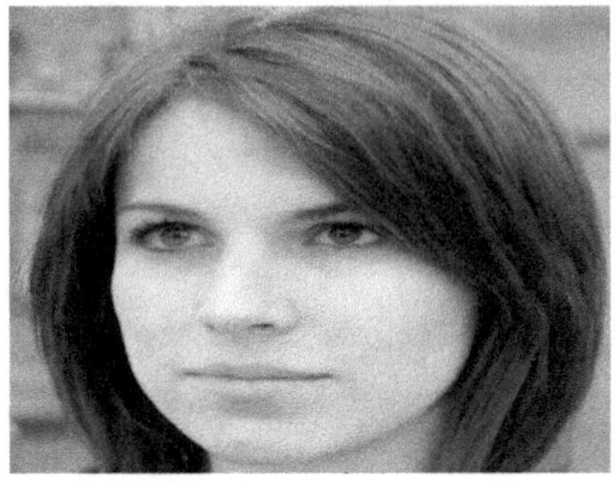

Jasmin W. Alcantara is not just an author but a devoted mom with a passion for health and well-being. As a dedicated mother, she understands the challenges that many individuals, especially moms, face on their journey towards weight loss and a healthier lifestyle.

Motivated by her own experiences and the desire to create a positive impact, Jasmin delves into the world of weight loss with a unique perspective. Her insights are not just rooted in research but grounded in the daily realities of balancing family life, personal well-being, and the pursuit of fitness goals.

Driven by a genuine commitment to help others navigate the often complex path of weight loss, Jasmin brings a compassionate and relatable approach to her writing. Through her work, she aims to empower moms and individuals alike, providing practical advice, motivational insights, and a roadmap for achieving sustainable health and fitness.

As a mom who understands the importance of time, Jasmin's strategies focus on practical and achievable steps that can be seamlessly integrated into busy lifestyles. Her writing reflects not only her knowledge but also her empathy, making her a trusted guide for those seeking a holistic approach to weight loss and overall wellness.

Jasmin W. Alcantara invites you to embark on a journey of self-discovery, resilience, and well-being. Through her words, she shares not just information but a genuine understanding of the challenges and triumphs that come with the pursuit of a healthier, happier life.

Losing Weight for Women

TABLE OF CONTENT

INTRODUCTION

Overview Of Weight Loss

What's Weight Loss?

Weight loss is the most widely recognized approach to subsiding your muscle versus fat. Exactly when you slip pounds, you're consuming further calories than you're consuming. This ought to be conceivable through a blend of diet and exercise.

What are the benefits of weight loss for women?

There are different benefits to losing weight for women. Advanced great Weight decrease can assist with culminating your general great and diminish your trouble of making consistent conditions practically equivalent to as heart snarling, stroke, type 2 diabetes, and a various quills of grievance. Extended energy conditions When you get more slender, you could have further energy and feel less depleted. Better tone-regard getting in shape can assist you with resting more straightforwardly pondering yourself and your appearance. Dropped pressure Weight decrease can assist with diminishing strain conditions.

Elevated place rest quality Weight decrease can assist you with snoozing more around night time.

How huge weight should women lose?

The Proportion of weight that women should lose depends upon their solitary circumstances. Anyway, most extremely outrageous women who are fat or fat should expect to lose 5-10% of their body weight.

What are sound approaches to slipping pounds?

There are different strong approaches to getting in shape. probably the voguish styles integrate Eating a sound eating authority A strong eating authority consolidates abundance of natural items, vegetables, and whole grains. It's in a manner essential to outline unwanted fats, reused food sources, and crude drinks. practicing regularly Pull out all the stops 30 beats of moderate-power practice most days of the week. Getting adequate rest most adults need around 7-8 hours of rest each night. Regulating Strain can provoke weight gain. Find sound approaches to supervising pressure, relative as yoga, assessment, or focusing profoundly on nature.

How are a few home exercises that ladies might get more fit?

There are many home exercises that ladies can do to get thinner. A few famous choices include:

Cardio: Cardio activities like running, swimming, and trekking can assist you with consuming calories and shed pounds.

Strength preparing: Strength preparing activities, for example, lifting loads or utilizing opposition groups can assist you with building muscle, which can assist you with consuming more calories very still.

Stop and go aerobic exercise (HIIT): HIIT is a kind of activity that shifts back and forth between short eruptions of extreme activity and times of rest. HIIT can be exceptionally compelling for consuming calories and shedding pounds.

What are a few ways to remain roused to shed pounds?

It tends to be hard to remain roused to get thinner. Here are a few hints to assist you with keeping focused:

Set forth sensible targets: Do whatever it takes not to endeavor to lose an inordinate measure of weight unreasonably quick. Set close to nothing, reachable targets and step by step increase them as you progress.

Find a genuinely strong organization: Find partners, family members, or a weight decrease social event to help you on your journey.

Reward yourself: Reward yourself for showing up at your targets. This will help you with remaining moves and make the cycle more lovely.

Do whatever it takes not to give up: There will be disasters in transit. Do whatever it takes not to leave yourself. Just keep on pushing ahead and you will at last show up at your targets.

In the current fast moving world, cutting out a valuable open door to focus on our prosperity and success can be a troublesome embrace. In any case, we acknowledge that managing your body should be open, profitable, and uniquely designed to your exceptional necessities. This book is your intensive manual for setting out on a pivotal trip towards a superior, more certain you, all from the comfort of your own home.

In the pages that follow, we will research the norms of weight loss, dive into the upsides of home activities, and give you realistic direction on the most ideal way to make your home a sanctuary for health. We need to connect with you to take care of your health cycle, not through tedious activity, community gatherings or patterns kept away from food, but instead through pragmatic and enchanting home activities.

Through this book, we'll help you with getting a handle on the fundamentals of weight loss, plan suitable rec center routine timetables, and foster a fair method for managing sustenance. You'll sort out some way to overcome troubles, stay roused, and acclaim your triumphs.

Weight loss can oftentimes have all the earmarks of being a startling test, especially when attacked with boundless eating routine examples and exercise regimens that ensure helpful arrangements. Regardless, really achieving a sound weight and staying aware of a well established trip should be spilling over with ecstasy and satisfaction.

The technique we outline in this book is focused on the likelihood that ease, convenience, and consistency are the keys to advance. We sort out the excellent necessities and stresses of women as they continue looking for a superior lifestyle, and we've fitted the substance to address those specific examinations.

Our book isn't just about shedding pounds; it's connected to building a more grounded, more grounded version of yourself. It's connected to gaining sureness and achieving a level of real thriving that further develops your life all around.

The journey to getting in shape and feeling your best doesn't have to be daunting. In light of everything, we'll guide you through sensible, convincing, and enchanting activities that can without a very remarkable stretch be coordinated into your regular everyday timetable. No necessity for exorbitant activity community enlistments or hours spent heading to health centers. We keep up with the idea that you ought to have the choice to work on your prosperity and health in the comfort of your own home.

Thus, how about we leave on this interesting experience together, as we investigate the universe of home exercises and find the force of adjusted sustenance. Prepare to venture out towards turning into the best and most joyful form of yourself. This excursion isn't just about shedding pounds; it's tied in with acquiring a dynamic, certain, and rejuvenated you.

When you get done with perusing, you'll have the information, instruments, and motivation expected to set out on your own home exercise venture. Thus, we should start this thrilling experience together and find the delights of accomplishing your optimal load such that suits your way of life and makes a positive, enduring effect on your wellbeing and prosperity.

CHAPTER 1

Setting Your Weight Loss Goals

As you keep searching for a superior, more certain version of yourself, the meaning of spreading out self-evident and reachable weight loss goals could never be more huge. These goals go about as your compass, guiding you through the complex yet remunerating journey of self-awareness. This segment plunges further into the most well-known approach to shaping your optimal self-insight and making targets that will draw in you to succeed.

Make sure you are ready:

Long term weight loss takes time and effort and a really long obligation. While you would prefer not to put off weight loss interminably, you should plan to carry out enduring upgrades to eating and development affinities. Present yourself the going with requests to help you with choosing your planning:

Am I energized to get more fit?

Am I too redirected by various pressures?

Do I include food as a method for adjusting to pressure?

Am I arranged to learn or use various approaches to adjust to pressure?

Do I truly need other assistance, either from buddies or specialists to administer pressure?

Am I prepared to change dietary examples?

Am I prepared to change activity affinities?

Do you have the valuable chance to spend on carrying out these enhancements?

Speak with your essential consideration doctor if you truly need help addressing stressors or sentiments that seem like blocks to your readiness. Exactly when you're ready, you'll find it more straightforward to characterize targets, stay committed and work on affinities.

Before characterizing your weight loss targets:

1. Contemplate your early phase: Begin by understanding your continuous weight, weight list (BMI), and muscle to fat proportion. This will give a benchmark to watching your turn of events.

2. Choose your motivation: Perceive the clarifications for your weight loss goals. Is it to deal with your prosperity, support your certainty, or update your genuine show? Understanding your motivation will help you with staying committed on your trip.

Defining Your Ideal Body

The idea of an ideal body is a profoundly private and extraordinary one. About accomplishing a condition of prosperity lines up with your own solace, wellbeing, and satisfaction, as opposed to adjusting to outer guidelines or ridiculous assumptions.

Chasing weight loss and a better way of life, characterizing your ideal body fills in as your North Star, directing your endeavors and rousing your excursion. Nonetheless, this idea goes past shallow appearances; it's tied in with making a dream of the best version of yourself regarding both physical and mental prosperity.

Past Style

Your ideal body ought to be an impression of your remarkable goals, inclinations, and generally speaking wellbeing targets. It's vital to move past society's thin magnificence guidelines and spotlight on what causes you to feel good, sure, and truly blissful.

Profound Prosperity

Consider how arriving at your ideal body can impact your profound state. Frequently, weight loss is related with expanded fearlessness, diminished tension, and worked on generally emotional wellness. Your ideal body ought to cause you to feel genuinely enabled.

Actual Ability

Your vision of your ideal body ought to likewise rotate around what your body can do, not exactly what it looks like. Consider the proactive tasks you need to participate in, whether it's climbing, moving, or essentially having the endurance for your everyday existence without exhaustion.

Wellbeing Driven Objectives

Focusing on wellbeing over simple style is a principal part of characterizing your optimal body. Weight loss isn't just about looking great; it's tied in with feeling better and decreasing the gamble of medical problems related with overabundance weight.

By and large Prosperity

Your ideal body ought to be one that advances prosperity, imperativeness, and life span. It's tied in with having the energy and versatility to lead a satisfying life and take on new difficulties.

Fitting to Your Necessities

Perceive that everybody's ideal body is exceptional, formed by individual inclinations and ailments. Your ideal could contrast from another person's, and that is entirely alright. Your objectives ought to be customized and as one with your particular necessities.

Setting Individual Goals

Characterizing your ideal body is a personal and engaging interaction. It includes setting individual targets that line up with your vision, and these objectives ought to go past numbers on a scale.

Center around Propensities

While it's fundamental to have weight-related objectives, it's similarly vital to zero in on the propensities that will assist you with accomplishing them. These propensities could incorporate eating more products of the soil, practicing routinely, or rehearsing care.

Non-Scale Triumphs

Recognize and celebrate non-scale triumphs, like expanded energy, better rest, further developed mind-set, and positive changes in your body creation. These triumphs are many times more characteristic of your general advancement than the number on the scale.

Characterizing your ideal body is definitely not a one-size-fits-all interaction. A profoundly private and extraordinary excursion envelops close to home prosperity, actual capacities, and a promise to a better, more dynamic you. As you set out on this excursion, remember that your vision of your ideal body ought to mirror your novel longings and goals, at last prompting a superior, really satisfying life.

A Comprehensive Viewpoint

While imagining your optimal body, consider what it can mean for your general wellbeing and health. Think about the enhancements in energy levels, everyday exercises, and your feeling of prosperity that can be accomplished by arriving at your optimal state.

Embracing Individualization

Embrace the possibility that everybody's ideal body contrasts, and there is no one size-fits-all methodology. Your ideal ought to mirror your inclinations, way of life, and goals, perceiving that is private and unmistakable.

In the mission to characterize your optimal body and leave on a fruitful weight loss venture, individualization is a significant and engaging idea. It recognizes that every individual is special, and what works for one may not work for another. Embracing individualization includes fitting your way to deal with your particular necessities, inclinations, and conditions.

Redoing Your Methodology

Perceiving and praising your independence is the groundwork of a feasible and fruitful weight loss venture.

Individual Inclinations

One critical part of individualization is recognizing your own inclinations. Your ideal body ought to be an impression of what makes you agreeable, blissful, and persuaded. Consider the kinds of activities you appreciate, the food varieties you love, and the schedules that best accommodate your way of life.

Way of life and Time Imperatives

Your regular routine and timetable assume a huge part in characterizing your optimal body. Think about your work, family, and different responsibilities. Your way to deal with weight loss ought to oblige these variables to guarantee that it's reasonable and maintainable.

Wellbeing Contemplations

Your wellbeing status and explicit necessities are basic components of individualization.

Prior Conditions

On the off chance that you have any prior medical issue, for example, diabetes or hypertension, your weight loss approach ought to line up with dealing with these circumstances. It might include talking with medical services experts to guarantee that your endeavors are protected and powerful.

Age and Phase of Life

Different life stages bring one of a kind contemplations. A weight loss plan for a lady in her 20s might vary essentially from that of a lady in her 50s. Individualization considers your age, hormonal changes, and any wellbeing worries that might be more pervasive at specific phases of life.

Self-Empathy

Embracing individualization likewise involves rehearsing self-sympathy. Comprehend that your process might have high points and low points, and that is ordinary. Try not to contrast yourself with others and spotlight on your own advancement and development.

In the realm of weight loss, one size doesn't fit all. Embracing individualization enables you to make an arrangement that suits your novel requirements, inclinations, and conditions. It's tied in with respecting your distinction and leaving on an excursion that prompts a better, more joyful, and more satisfied you. Recollect that the way to your ideal body is an individual one, and the objective is extraordinarily yours to characterize.

Creating Realistic and Achievable Goals

Whenever you've illustrated your ideal body, the following critical step is to put forth objectives that are both common sense and achievable. These objectives will act as your achievements, keeping you propelled and on target all through your weight loss venture.

Returning to Brilliant Objectives

The Brilliant (Explicit, Quantifiable, Attainable, Important, Time-bound) system remains your dearest companion in creating powerful objectives.

Specific: Drill down your objectives to exact goals. Create some distance from dubious thoughts like "get fit" and spotlight on particulars, for example, "shed 25 pounds."

Measurable: Guarantee your objectives are quantifiable so you can keep tabs on your development and praise your achievements.

Achievable: Objectives ought to be tested however inside your compass. Setting targets that are too aggressive can prompt dissatisfaction and debilitation.

Relevance: Your objectives ought to orchestrate with your way of life, values, and long haul desires.

Time-bound: Lay out a sensible time period for your objectives. For instance, "shed 25 pounds in eight months."

Present moment and Long haul Objectives

Think about both present moment and long haul objectives. Momentary objectives can assist you with remaining inspired and gathering speed, while long haul objectives give the master plan. An illustration of a momentary objective could be "practice for 30 minutes each day in the current week," while a drawn out objective may be "arrive at my optimal load in a year."

Momentary Objectives

Momentary objectives act as building blocks. They assist you with gaining ground rapidly and keep up with your inspiration. Models incorporate intending to practice for 30 minutes each day in the current week or integrating more vegetables into your dinners.

Long haul Objectives

Long haul objectives give a higher perspective. They address your general goals, like arriving at your optimal load in no less than a year or finishing a half-long distance race in a half year. These are the yearnings that drive your excursion.

Observe Each Triumph

Try not to misjudge the force of praising your accomplishments, no matter what their size. Recognizing your advancement, regardless of how little, is fundamental for supporting your responsibility and sustaining the fervor for the excursion ahead.

As you start your weight loss venture, recollect that all around created, attainable objectives structure the bedrock of your prosperity. Your unmistakable ideal body and Savvy objectives will be your directing stars, guiding you towards a better, more sure, and more joyful you.

CHAPTER 2

Understanding Weight Loss

Prior to leaving on a weight loss venture, it's vital to handle the essentials of how weight loss functions. This information will enable you to pursue informed choices and set sensible assumptions for your change. In this part, we'll investigate the connection between calories, digestion, and diet, revealing insight into the science behind weight loss.

What You Can Expect While Getting thinner

On the off chance that you've at any point attempted another prevailing fashion diet, you understand what a crazy thrill ride of an excursion it very well may be. Before you start your next weight loss arrangement, get to know these phases of weight loss.

Information is power! Being familiar with the actual phases of weight loss can make it more straightforward for you to get past the intense ones and arrive at your ultimate objective — long haul, sound weight loss.

Fat Misfortune versus Weight loss

Before we get to the phases of weight loss, understanding the distinctions between fat misfortune and weight loss is significant. They're not similar!

Consider weight loss the all-encompassing term for the numbers on the scale going down. Where it gets befuddling is that weight loss isn't guaranteed to cause fat misfortune. For the vast majority, while getting thinner, fat misfortune is a definitive objective. Yet, when you initially begin confining your calories, you get more fit, not fat.

It's basic to know the distinction so that when the numbers on the scale slow down or you see enormous changes everyday, you know that that is simply typical weight loss. With weight loss, you're seeing changes in how much water your body holds, the amount you ate the other day, and waste you presently can't seem to empty.

Weight loss is typical while eating less junk food, yet your definitive objective ought to be to acquire or keep up with your muscles and lose fat. To energize fat misfortune rather than simply weight loss, you ought to eat a lot of protein while making a calorie shortfall in your eating routine and expanding your active work levels. To ensure you're losing fat, put resources into a scale that actions your muscle to fat ratio content.

5 Phases of Weight Loss

During your weight loss venture, you're probably going to go through various stages and stages. While there's a standard example of weight loss stages, you could likewise find that you go through a portion of the stages on different occasions and could skirt a few phases.
As you start your weight loss venture, here are the actual phases of weight loss you ought to hope to go through.

1. The Special first night

The principal period of a weight loss venture is about hopefulness, that is the reason we refer to it as "The Special first night Stage". Your weight loss plan is brilliant and sparkly and new. It appears to be attainable and not excessively prohibitive. You have lots of inspiration and are eager to get everything rolling.

In the beginning phases of the wedding trip stage, you're cooking at home, setting up your dinners, pursuing solid decisions, and normal exercises. You're 100 percent committed.

The most amazing aspect? You're probably in any event, seeing some development on the scale. This is an incredible stage, and an extraordinary spot to begin your weight loss venture. Sadly, it doesn't last forever. Life and reality begin to disrupt everything.

Quick Weight loss

During this first phase of weight loss, you'll see that it seems like the pounds are simply tumbling off. During the initial four to about a month and a half of your weight loss venture, you'll shed pounds and you'll lose it rapidly.

However, it's essential to remember that during the principal phase of weight loss , a significant part of the weight you're losing is from water. As you decrease your calorie consumption, your body starts to consume its abundance of glycogen stores, which are put away in your liver and muscles.

While this outcomes in a more modest number on the scale, you're not really losing (much) fat during this stage. When your body has consumed its overabundant glycogen stores, it can start to consume fat. This is known as ketosis.

Your weight loss is impacted by the structure of your eating routine, the quantity of calories you consume, your age, sex, beginning weight, and actual work.

Try not to allow this to put you down. Watch those numbers go down and utilize that as fuel to keep inspiring you into the following body phases of weight loss.

2. Rude awakening: More slow Weight loss

For any individual who has evaluated another eating regimen, you know how difficult the rude awakening is. You're doing great arranging your dinners, keeping away from the inexpensive food and bite machine, and afterward genuine interrupts. You get up late or your child has a crisis and your feast plan escapes whack. You think of yourself as all over town, eager and tired. So you drive-through some place for a helpful feast.

This little thing can crash your whole mental arrangement for your new eating routine. It can require several days or even seven days to get back ready assuming you at any point do. This psychological blockage and genuineness can slow your weight loss objectives.

More slow weight loss is an ordinary, normal stage in the phases of weight loss.

Slow Weight loss

During this period of slower weight loss, you might see that you're shedding weight all the more leisurely and you might arrive at a weight loss level where you're proceeding to eat a confined calorie diet however aren't losing any weight whatsoever.

This is typical.

But on the other hand, it's extremely baffling. This phase of your fat misfortune excursion can be intellectually and genuinely burdening. Your inspiration is winding down and everything appears to be only a tad bit harder.

Weight loss levels can be brought about by excessively prohibitive eating regimens that are too challenging to even consider adhering to and metabolic variations, where your body adjusts to the lower calorie intake.

While picking an eating routine, it's critical to track down something that accommodates your way of life and can be a super durable change that you can stay with.

While the progressions on the scale come all the more leisurely during this stage, it's truly a truly significant stage. During this sluggish weight loss stage, you're really losing fat, which is the objective.

One thing to look out for: hunger. During this stage, you might feel more ravenous, more regularly. Search for high-protein tidbits and dinners to assist you with feeling full longer.

3. Battle the Level: **DO. NOT. GET. DISCOURAGED.**

The third condition of weight loss comes in whenever you've been confining your calories for a really long time. You've previously gone through a profound exciting ride with numerous misfortunes and mix-ups. This phase of your weight loss venture is tied in with finding balance and not getting deterred.

During this stage, you could observe that you're more predictable with picking quality feast choices and getting exercise. You're adhering to your feast plan more often than not and controlling your bits. You've constructed an underpinning of solid propensities. What's more, you've additionally understood that the weight loss interaction will take time and exertion.

Building solid propensities is troublesome, however this stage is about maintainability and inspiration. Routine can get exhausting, so it means a lot to track down ways of keeping yourself intrigued. This weight loss venture is long haul. Finding little, sound prizes en route can help you from getting deterred and surrendering.

4. Genuine Way of life Change

In the fourth phase of weight loss, you'll find that your propensities have become so profoundly imbued that you never again contemplate them. You anticipate your week by week feast arranging meeting, you ache for protein-rich, vegetable-weighty dinners, and your companions never again question your request when you go out to eat.

Congratulations!!

You're not simply consuming less calories, you've made a valid, maintainable change to your way of life and dietary patterns. This is an extraordinary stage to be in. Your eating regimen feels regular and manageable. You comprehend your desires and how to satisfy them without indulging.

While this can be a profoundly fulfilling phase of your weight loss venture, it won't endure forever. You could swing to and fro between various stages. That is typical! You want to construct propensities for valid, extremely durable fat misfortune.

5. Keeping up with Weight loss

The last actual phase of weight loss is keeping up with your weight loss. With many eating regimens, you're urged to deny yourself to rapidly get more fit. The disadvantage to these kinds of diets is that you're bound to yo and recover the weight you've lost.

Keeping up with your weight loss ought to be similarly as essential to you as getting thinner. Weight loss upkeep isn't just about eating in an unexpected way, it's tied in with changing your way of behaving.

The following are a couple of procedures to help you keep up with and complete the phases of weight loss.

Keep quality food available. The food you see is the food you're probably going to eat. Purchase good food choices, for example, products of the soil and keep them where you can see them, on the counter in a bowl, and unmistakably put away in the cooler. Extra focuses: set up your leafy foods so you have in and out snacks.

Keep away from handled food sources. Handled food varieties are by and large higher in calories, fat, and sugar. By staying away from handled food varieties, you will naturally float towards entire, quality food varieties. Increment protein admission. Protein assists with keeping you feeling full longer. At the point when you center around eating protein-rich dinners, you'll get full and remain full. This assists you with staying away from the munchies and going after a bite.

Track and self-screen. Keeping a food diary and following your activity can assist you to self-screen and increment your mindfulness of ways of behaving and what they mean for your weight loss.

Find development that satisfies you. Actual work is a critical piece of weight loss support. Assuming you have found development and exercise that satisfies you, that will make it almost certain that you'll make it happen. Having different exercises can likewise help. You can go to the rec center now and again, take yoga classes, have solo dance gatherings, and go for strolls around your area. With choices, you can move consistently and not get exhausted.

Make a pressure on the executives' plan. Stress is a central point in weight loss and weight loss upkeep. At the point when we feel anxious, a considerable lot of us go after solace food varieties, which will generally be profoundly handled or brimming with carbs and fat. Your pressure the executives plan ought to incorporate solid ways of managing your pressure.

Sleep! Many individuals fail to remember that rest is a fundamental piece of wellbeing. At the point when we need rest or keep awake until late, our body longs for speedy energy sources, which incorporate carbs and sugars. By getting a lot of rest, your body is very much refreshed and desires will be restricted.

The weight loss interaction can be slow and monotonous. You could quickly return and forward between the various phases of weight loss, which can be exceptionally personal.

While the beginning phases of weight loss can be loaded up with trust and accomplishment while you're rapidly getting thinner, the following stages, where weight loss dials back and you could hit a level, can baffle. Tracking down basic reassurance and ways of changing your way of behaving can make it more straightforward to traverse every one of the phases of weight loss.

Calories and Weight: The Fundamental Connection

Understanding the association among calories and weight is major in your weight decrease adventure. Calories are the units of energy found in the food sources and beverages we finish, and they expect a pivotal part in concluding our body weight.

Caloric Confirmation versus Utilization

The indispensable rule to make sense of is the agreement between the calories you consume and the calories you consume. It's often implied as the "caloric condition."

Caloric Affirmation

- Calories finished come from the food sources and refreshments you ingest. This integrates starches, fats, proteins, and beverages.

- Different food sources have different calorie contents. For example, a gram of fat contains a bigger number of calories than a gram of carbs or protein.

- It's basic to keep a fair eating schedule, as the idea of calories moreover impacts your overall prosperity and success.

Caloric Use

- The calories you devour various means, including your basal metabolic rate (BMR), dynamic work, and the thermic effect of food (TEF).

- BMR tends to the calories your body needs to do major jobs like breathing, overseeing temperature, and staying aware of organ ability.

- Genuine work, including action and everyday turn of events, can on a very basic level influence the calories you consume.

- TEF addresses the calories your body utilizes handling, charming, and using the food you eat.

The Calorie deficiency

To shed pounds, you should make a calorie deficiency. This implies you consume a bigger number of calories than you consume.

Weight loss

- At the point when you reliably keep a calorie deficiency, your body begins utilizing put away energy (normally fat) to compensate for the shortage.

- These outcomes in weight loss over the long haul.

Feasible Weight loss

- Making a humble calorie deficiency is vital to accomplishing reasonable weight loss.

- Outrageous calorie limitation can prompt muscle misfortune and dietary lacks, which are counterproductive to your objectives.

Past the Numbers

It's essential to perceive that not all calories are made equivalent. The nature of calories, as well as the supplements they give, assumes a critical part in your general wellbeing.

Supplement Thick Food varieties

- Food varieties that are plentiful in fundamental supplements, like nutrients, minerals, fiber, and cell reinforcements, can uphold your wellbeing and weight loss objectives.

Supplement thick food sources are plentiful in fundamental supplements like nutrients, minerals, fiber, and cancer prevention agents while being somewhat low in calories. Remembering these food varieties for your eating regimen can assist you with accomplishing your weight loss and generally wellbeing objectives. Here are a few models:

1. *Salad Greens:* Spinach, kale, Swiss chard, and collard greens are loaded with nutrients and minerals, especially vitamin K, vitamin A, and folate.

2. *Berries:* Blueberries, strawberries, and raspberries are stacked with cancer prevention agents, nutrients, and fiber. They're brilliant for your general wellbeing.

3. Nuts and Seeds: Almonds, pecans, flaxseeds, and chia seeds give solid fats, fiber, and various fundamental supplements.

4. Salmon: Greasy fish like salmon are wealthy in omega-3 unsaturated fats, which are useful for heart wellbeing and generally prosperity.

5. Legumes: Beans, lentils, and chickpeas are high in protein, fiber, nutrients, and minerals. They are astounding wellsprings of plant-based protein.

6. Entire Grains: Oats, quinoa, earthy colored rice, and entire wheat pasta give complex starches, fiber, and a scope of supplements.

7. Fruits: Apples, oranges, and pears are tasty as well as give fundamental nutrients, fiber, and cancer prevention agents.

8. Greek Yogurt: Low-fat or sans fat Greek yogurt is high in protein and probiotics, which are perfect for stomach wellbeing.

9. Eggs: Eggs are a wellspring of excellent protein, nutrients, and minerals. They can be important for a reasonable eating routine.

10. Yams: These give a decent wellspring of mind boggling sugars, fiber, and beta-carotene, which is changed over into vitamin A in the body.

11. Broccoli: This vegetable is plentiful in nutrients C and K, fiber, and different cell reinforcements.

12. Ringer Peppers: They are an extraordinary wellspring of L-ascorbic acid and fiber while being low in calories.

13. Lean Meats: Skinless poultry, lean cuts of meat, and pork flank offer protein and fundamental supplements without overabundance fat.

14. Dairy: Low-fat or sans fat dairy items like milk and yogurt are great wellsprings of calcium and protein.

15. Avocado: Avocado is a sound wellspring of monounsaturated fats, fiber, and a few nutrients, including vitamin K, E, and C.

Remembering these supplement thick food sources for your eating routine can assist you with meeting your wholesome necessities while dealing with your weight and advancing in general prosperity.

Adjusted Nourishment

- A fair eating routine that gives every one of the fundamental supplements guarantees your body works ideally and upholds generally speaking prosperity.

Understanding the basic association among calories and weight is the most vital phase in your weight loss venture. It enables you to go with informed decisions about your eating regimen, exercise, and in general way of life. By making a reasonable calorie deficiency through a decent methodology, you can accomplish your weight loss objectives while focusing on your wellbeing and prosperity.

Metabolism and Diet

Understanding the complex connection among digestion and diet is pivotal for improving your general wellbeing, energy levels, and weight. Your digestion goes about as your body's motor, deciding how productively it processes and uses the energy obtained from the food varieties you eat.

The Rudiments of Digestion

Digestion incorporates the mind boggling set of synthetic cycles that happen inside your body to keep up with life. It includes two essential parts:

Basal Metabolic Rate (BMR)

- BMR addresses the quantity of calories your body needs very still to keep up with essential physiological capabilities like breathing, course, and cell creation.
- Factors affecting BMR incorporate age, orientation, body creation, and hereditary qualities.

Actual work and Thermic Impact of Food (TEF)

- Actual work, including activity and day to day development, adds to the calories your body consumes.
- TEF addresses the energy consumed during processing, assimilation, and digestion of food. Certain food sources require more energy for processing, adding to TEF.

The Impact of Diet on Digestion

Your eating routine assumes a huge part in molding your digestion. Certain dietary decisions can influence the rate at which your body processes and uses energy.

Protein-Rich Food varieties

- Protein has a higher thermic impact contrasted with fats and sugars. This implies your body exhausts more energy processing and utilizing protein, adding to calorie consumption.

- Counting lean wellsprings of protein like chicken, fish, tofu, and vegetables can uphold a sound digestion.

Fiber-Rich Food varieties

- High-fiber food varieties, like organic products, vegetables, and entire grains, add to generally speaking stomach related wellbeing as well as give a sensation of completion, possibly decreasing by and large calorie consumption.

Adjusted Supplement Admission

- Consuming an even eating regimen that incorporates various supplements is fundamental for supporting general metabolic wellbeing.

- Fundamental nutrients and minerals go through a different eating regimen that assume urgent parts in the biochemical cycles that direct digestion.

Hydration

- Remaining sufficiently hydrated is essential for metabolic cycles. Water is engaged with various biochemical responses, including those connected with energy digestion.

Dinner Timing and Recurrence

When and how frequently you eat can likewise impact your digestion.

Normal Feasts

- Reliable, adjusted feasts and snacks over the course of the day can assist with keeping up with stable glucose levels and backing a consistent digestion.

Breakfast Significance

- Having a nutritious breakfast can launch your digestion after the short-term fasting time frame, giving energy to the day.

Actual work and Digestion

Actual work is a powerful powerhouse of digestion:

Strength Preparing

- Fabricating and keeping up with fit muscle through strength preparing can improve BMR, as muscle tissue requires more energy very still than fat tissue.

Cardiovascular Activity

- Cardiovascular activities add to calorie use during the movement and can emphatically affect by and large metabolic wellbeing.

Understanding the exchange among digestion and diet engages you to settle on informed decisions that help your general prosperity. By sustaining your body with a reasonable eating regimen, including digestion supporting supplements, remaining hydrated, and consolidating normal active work, you can enhance your metabolic wellbeing and advance a better, more vivacious you.

A Wholistic Approach

It's critical to recognize that effective weight loss is certainly not a simple numbers game; it's likewise complicatedly connected to by and large wellbeing and prosperity. Finding some kind of harmony between a sensible calorie deficiency, supplementing thick food varieties, and normal active work is the way into a practical and sound weight loss venture.

As you dive into the universe of weight loss, this comprehension of the center standards gives the compass you want to explore the multifaceted landscape, settle on very much educated decisions, and embrace a thorough methodology that prompts a lighter you, yet a better and more lively you.

CHAPTER 3

Preparing Your Home Workout Space: Creating a Fitness Haven

Setting up a devoted and welcoming home exercise space is vital to keeping a steady work-out daily practice. Whether you have an entire room or simply a corner in excess, this is the way to change it into a wellness shelter.

1. Pick the Right Area

Investigating your home and choosing the ideal place to set up your home rec center is a fundamental undertaking you mustn't mess with. To come to the best choice, think about the accompanying things:

Accessible space

Roof level

Ventilation and wind current

Normal light

Availability

Security and interruptions

Flooring

Primary uprightness

Capacity and associations

Commotion contemplations

A fitting space upholds the appropriate position of hardware, gives adequate space to development, guarantees great ventilation and lighting, and advances the center by limiting interruptions. Hence, smart space choice sets the establishment for a favorable climate that supports customary activity and helps in accomplishing your wellness objectives.

2. Accumulate Fundamental Gear

You needn't bother with an exercise center of gear. Begin with the fundamentals:

- Practice Mat: Gives solace to floor activities and yoga.

- Opposition Groups: Adaptable for strength preparing and extending.

- Hand weights or Iron weights: Pick loads appropriate for your wellness level.

- Work out with Rope: Fantastic for cardio exercises.

- Security Ball: Incredible for center activities.

- Reflect: Assists with structure and inspiration.

3. Set up legitimate lightning

Lighting influences perceivability as well as the mood of your space, which can fundamentally impact your inspiration and energy levels. Begin by expanding regular light as it advances a better climate and lifts state of mind. For regions lacking regular light, utilize fake lighting in a calculated manner. Utilize splendid, elevated lights for focused energy exercises to guarantee wellbeing, while gentler, movable lights can make a quieting environment for exercises like yoga or extending.

Furthermore, consider task lighting for explicit regions, for example, a perusing light by your treadmill for the people who like to peruse during their cardio meetings. Generally, very much arranged lighting hoists your exercise space from being absolutely useful to an intriguing, rousing sanctuary that upgrades your wellness process.

4. Make an Inspirational Environment

Make your exercise space motivating:

- Add Plants: Plant life can upgrade the feel and further develop air quality.

- Adorn with Inspirational Statements: Encircle yourself with positive updates.

Invigorating Tones: Consolidate colors that support energy and inspiration:

Brilliant Shades: Select energetic varieties like red, orange, or yellow to make an enthusiastic environment.

Emphasize Wall: Consider painting one wall in a stimulating tone or utilizing strip-and-stick backdrop for a transitory and customized touch.

5. Arrange Your Space

Keep your exercise region clean and open:

- Capacity Arrangements: Use containers, racks, or cupboards to conveniently store hardware.

- Open Space: Guarantee there's adequate space for dynamic developments without hindrances.

6. Connecting with Visuals

Use visuals to invigorate inspiration:

Wellness Banners or Craftsmanship: Enhance your space with pictures that feature the exercises you love or try to succeed in.

Vision Board: Make a dream board with wellness objectives, uplifting statements, and pictures that address your goals.

Individual Accomplishments Show: Grandstand your wellness achievements, like awards, declarations, or photographs of wellness achievements.

7. Set Up Innovation

Use tech to upgrade your exercises:

Fortifying Music

Set the vibe with an inspiring soundtrack:

Sound Framework: Put resources into great quality speakers to partake in your #1 exercise tunes.

Organized Playlists: Make playlists with high-energy tunes that siphon you up and keep you moving.

Assortment of Classifications: Stir up classifications to match different exercise states of mind, from peppy cardio meetings to quieting stretches.

- Wellness Applications: Keep tabs on your development and remain propelled.

8. Customize Your Space

Adding components that mirror your character and inclinations can upgrade inspiration and pleasure during exercises. Maybe, it's banners of your wellness symbols, music speakers for your exercise playlist, or a corner for post-exercise unwinding with your #1 book. Integrating components connected with your leisure activities, or tones that empower or alleviate you, can make the space seriously welcoming.

This tailor-made climate suits your stylish preferences as well as fills in as a steady sign of your wellness objectives, making your gym routine more tomfoolery and successful. All things considered, in your customized home rec center, you're not simply working out, you're flourishing.

In building your home exercise center, you've made a space that genuinely mirrors your wellness objectives and individual inclinations. It's something beyond an exercise space, it's a sanctuary custom-made to your novel process towards better wellbeing. Keep in mind, the cycle doesn't end here; proceed to adjust and develop your wellness safe house as you overcome an endless flow of objectives.

9. Center around Security and Solace

Most importantly, guarantee that your home rec center has sufficient open space to securely oblige your activities and developments. A messiness free climate forestalls exercise related wounds. Consider putting resources into a padded deck that gives soundness during exercises and decreases the gamble of strain or injury.

For solace, think about the temperature in your exercise region. Introducing a fan or a warmer can keep an agreeable temperature consistently. Your exercise region ought to likewise have sufficient lighting to guarantee perceivability. Ultimately, utilize ergonomic hardware intended for usability and limiting strain. By focusing on wellbeing and solace, you can make an exercise space that energizes predictable use and supports your wellness process.

Think about Multi-Practical Furnishings

On the off chance that your exercise space imparts a space to different capabilities:

- Foldable Gear: Put resources into gear that can be effectively put away.
- Convertible Furnishings: Pick things that fill a double need, similar to an exercise seat that can likewise be a seating region.

Making a devoted home exercise space is an interest in your wellbeing and prosperity. By organizing a climate that lines up with your inclinations, you'll be more spurred and steady in your work-out daily schedule, at last prompting a better and more joyful you.

CHAPTER 4

Warm-Up and Stretching: Priming Your Body for Exercise

Prior to jumping into your exercise, committing time to a legitimate warm-up and extending routine is essential for setting up your body, forestalling wounds, and streamlining your presentation. Here is a manual to assist you with making a successful warm-up and extending a meeting.

Significance of Warm-Up

Setting up Your Body for Activity

A legitimate warm-up isn't simply an introduction to your exercise; a fundamental part makes way for ideal execution and helps protect your body from expected wounds. Here's the reason a warm-up is fundamental prior to participating in actual work:

1. Expanded Blood Stream:

A warm-up continuously builds your pulse and blood dissemination, conveying oxygen and supplements to your muscles. This sets them up for the expanded requests of activity.

2. Further developed Muscle Temperature:

Warm muscles are more malleable and responsive. As your internal heat level ascents during a warm-up, your muscles become more adaptable, decreasing the gamble of strains and tears.

3. Improved Joint Adaptability:

Controlled powerful developments during a warm-up increment the scope of movement in your joints. This is significant for exercises that include bowing, curving, and turning.

4. Actuation of Sensory system:

A warm-up invigorates your sensory system, improving the association between your mind and muscles. This superior neuromuscular capability brings about better coordination and responsiveness during exercise.

5. Mental Readiness:

Truly setting up your body additionally primes your brain for the impending action. It helps shift your concentration to the exercise, advancing fixation and lessening the gamble of interruptions.

6. Injury Counteraction:

A progressive warm-up permits your body to adjust to expanded pressure slowly, bringing down the gamble of wounds. Cold muscles and joints are more inclined to strains and wounds.

7. Expanded Proficiency of Energy Frameworks:

The warm-up signals your body to move from a resting state to a functioning one, improving the productivity of your energy frameworks. This guarantees a smoother change into higher-force work out.

8. Quicker Muscle Constriction and Unwinding:

A warm-up speeds up the pace of muscle constriction and unwinding. This speedy reaction is fundamental for exercises requiring quick developments or shifts in course.

9. Further developed Oxygen Conveyance:

Expanded blood stream from the warm-up guarantees that your muscles get a more effective inventory of oxygen. This is imperative for supporting perseverance during vigorous exercises.

10. Post-Exercise Recuperation:

A legitimate warm-up assists your body with changing all the more easily from the raised force of activity to the resting state. This can add to a more agreeable and powerful recuperation.

11. Transformation to Exercise Climate:

On the off chance that you're progressing from a stationary state to active work, a warm-up permits your body to adjust to the natural circumstances, like temperature and moistness.

12. Long haul Adaptability and Portability:

Ordinary warm-ups add to working on long haul adaptability and versatility. After some time, this can upgrade your general wellness and lessen the gamble of old enough related solidness.

Integrating an insightful warm-up into your wellness routine is a little venture that yields huge returns. It not just readies your body for the quick requests of activity yet in addition adds to your drawn out wellbeing and prosperity. Making the warm-up a non-debatable piece of your routine is a brilliant and proactive way to deal with actual work.

Stretching: Improving Adaptability and Scope of Movement

1. Static Extending:

Hold each stretch for 15-30 seconds, zeroing in on significant muscle gatherings. Incorporate stretches for:

- Hamstrings: Go after your toes while situated or standing.

- Quadriceps: Pull your foot toward your bum.

- Chest: Catch your hands behind your back and fix your arms.

- Shoulders: Tenderly force one arm across your chest.

2. Dynamic Extending:

Integrate controlled, smooth motions through a full scope of movement. Models incorporate leg swings, arm circles, and strolling lurches.

3. Proprioceptive Neuromuscular Assistance (PNF):

High level extending procedure including a mix of compression and unwinding. Accomplice helped PNF extending can be viable for expanding adaptability.

4. Yoga or Pilates Moves:

Incorporate yoga postures or Pilates practices that accentuate adaptability and equilibrium. These can likewise advance mental concentration and unwinding.

5. Froth Rolling:

Utilize a froth roller on unambiguous muscle gatherings to deliver pressure and upgrade adaptability. Center around regions inclined to snugness, like calves, quadriceps, and upper back.

6. Ballistic Extending (Mindfulness):

Ballistic extending includes bobbing or swinging developments. While it can increase adaptability, it ought to be drawn nearer with mindfulness to stay away from injury. It's for the most part suggested for people with a deep rooted adaptability base.

7. Calf Raises and Toe Contacts:

Perform calf raises to extend and fortify the lower leg muscles. Consolidate this with toe contacts to draw in the hamstrings and lower back. Hold the stretches momentarily to keep up with control.

8. Neck Stretches:

Incorporate delicate neck stretches to deliver strain. Gradually slant your head to each side, forward, and in reverse, holding each stretch for a couple of moments.

9. Butterfly Stretch:

Sit with the bottoms of your feet together, permitting your knees to fall toward the floor. Hold your feet and tenderly press your knees toward the ground to extend the inward thighs.

10. Hip Flexor Stretch:

Bow on one knee while broadening the other leg forward. Tenderly push your hips forward to extend the hip flexors. Change sides to target the two legs.

11. Kid's Posture:

From a bowing position, sit out of sorts and arrive at your arms forward. This stretch focuses on the lower back, hips, and shoulders.

Tips for a Compelling Warm-Up and Extending Meeting:

Inhale Profoundly: Breathe in profoundly before each stretch and breathe out as you extend the stretch. Profound breathing advances unwinding and adaptability.

Abstain from Skipping: While performing static stretches, abstain from bobbing, as it can prompt muscle strain. All things considered, center around a steady, controlled stretch.

Continuous Movement: Begin with lighter power and slowly increment the force of your warm-up.

Individualized Approach: Tailor your warm-up and extending routine to your particular exercise and individual necessities.

Mind-Body Association: Utilize this opportunity to plan for your exercise, zeroing in on your objectives and goals intellectually.

Consistency: Make warm-up and extend a steady piece of your daily practice. Standard extending meetings add to long haul adaptability. Hold back nothing 10-15 minutes of extending a few times each week.

Pay attention to Your Body: Focus on how your body answers every development. On the off chance that something doesn't feel right, adjust or skip it. Stretch to the mark of gentle inconvenience, not torment. On the off chance that you feel torment, you might be pushing excessively hard.

By integrating a balanced warm-up and extending routine into your exercise routine, you set up for a more powerful and charming activity experience. It's an interest in your general wellness, forestalling wounds and advancing long haul adaptability and versatility.

CHAPTER 5

Effective Home Workouts: Maximizing Fitness in Your Living Space

Making a compelling home exercise routine permits you to focus on your wellbeing and wellness without the requirement for a rec center. Here is a manual for assist you with making effective home exercises:

1. Evaluate Your Objectives:

Characterize your wellness objectives, whether it's weight loss, muscle conditioning, working on cardiovascular wellbeing, or a mix. Tailor your home exercises to line up with your targets.

2. Make a Predictable Timetable:

Lay out a customary exercise timetable to construct a daily practice. Consistency is key for accomplishing and keeping up with wellness objectives.

3. Pick Different Activities:

Integrate a blend of cardio, strength preparing, adaptability, and equilibrium. Assortment keeps your exercises drawing in and targets various parts of wellness.

4. Cardiovascular Activities:

Settle on exercises that hoist your pulse. Models incorporate hopping jacks, high knees, jumping rope, or even dance exercises. No hardware required.

5. Strength Preparing:

Use bodyweight practices like squats, thrusts, push-ups, and boards. Incorporate family things as stopgap loads for added opposition.

6. HIIT (Extreme cardio exercise):

Consolidate short eruptions of extraordinary activity with times of rest. This productive technique consumes calories and lifts digestion.

7. Yoga and Pilates:

Further develop adaptability and center strength with yoga or Pilates schedules. Follow online recordings or applications for directed meetings.

8. High-intensity aerobics:

Make circuits joining various activities. Play out each activity for a set time frame or number of reiterations prior to moving to the following:

Jump from one side to another as you stand with your feet together.

- Bounce starting with one side then onto the next evenly, landing gently with your knees bowed.

For balance, draw your center line.

On Deck, Jacks:

Place your hands under your shoulders as you begin in the board position.

Maintain your board position as you bounce your feet back together and out wide.

Control your development while maintaining a tight center.

Boxing Swing:

Keep your feet roughly shoulder-width apart as you stand.

- Move your feet while running slowly.

Maintain your current speed while moving quickly.

Fast Feet:

- Stand with your feet about hip width separated.

Tap your feet on the ground quickly as you move quickly.

Maintain a light, alert, and mindful state while attracting your middle.

Preceding starting the circuit, make it a highlight warm up and chill off. Feel free to change the exercises as demonstrated by your tendencies and health level, changing the power and length. Bodyweight cardio circuits are a versatile and fundamental choice for an activity that gets your heart pumping wherever and whenever you want.

9. Step and stair workouts:

Cardio workouts can be done on stairs or step-ups. This simple but effective exercise targets your legs and raises your heart rate.

10. Tabata Activities:

Follow the Tabata's format: Repeat the centered energy practice for four minutes, then take a 10-second break. This can be utilized with various activities.

11. Make Activities Work for Your Situation Right Now:

Exercises ought to be altered in accordance with the available space. Without forfeiting plentifulness, it is feasible to adjust headways to suit areas that are less meddlesome.

12. Consolidate days off for recuperation:

Permit your body time to recuperate. On recuperation days, practice yoga, gentle walking, or stretching to increase adaptability and relaxation.

13. Set forward Reasonable Targets:

Distribute attainable milestones and each incremental step toward turning progress. Celebrate small victories to keep yourself going.

14. Eat well and drink enough water:

Support your exercises with legitimate hydration and a reasonable eating regimen. Meals high in nutrients contribute to fitness and overall health.

15. Form over repetition should come first:

To avoid injuries, focus on proper form. Quality developments are more advantageous than hurrying through reiterations with unfortunate structure.

16. Include friends or family members:

Transform exercises into a common action. Make it a social and enjoyable experience by inviting family members or roommates to join.

17. Remain Adaptable with Exercise Plans:

Be versatile. Keep alternate workout plans on hand in case of busy days or unforeseen changes in life.

It takes creativity, commitment, and a little bit of experimentation to create effective home workouts. As your fitness improves, modify your routine to fit your preferences and gradually push yourself. With devotion and consistency, your living space can turn into a flourishing center for accomplishing and keeping up with your wellness objectives.

Strength Preparing for Home Exercises: Building Power Anywhere

Strength training at home can be done with little equipment and be effective. A comprehensive guide to developing a robust home strength training program is provided here:

1. Evaluate Your Space and Equipment:

- Determine the equipment and space available at home.

- Fundamental hardware like free weights, opposition groups, and a security ball can upgrade your exercises.

2. Select exercises for the entire body:

- Select activities that connect with numerous muscle gatherings.

- Models incorporate squats, thrusts, push-ups, and pushes.

3. Establish a routine:

- Create a routine that is well-balanced and works all of the major muscle groups.

- Incorporate chest area, lower body, and center activities.

4. Warm-Up Properly:

- Start with five to ten minutes of light cardio (jumping jacks, stationary jogging).

- Follow with dynamic stretches to set up your muscles.

5. Opposition Band Exercises:

Pull-Apart Bands:

- Hold an obstruction band before you with arms extended.

- Engage your upper back by tearing the band apart.

Posterior Leg Raises:

- Adhere a bandage to your ankles.

- Against the resistance, raise one leg sideways.

Seating in the Row:

- Circle the band around a solid anchor.

- Row the band in your direction as you sit with your legs out.

6. Include Advancements:

- Consistently reconsider your solidarity and add movements to your activities.

- This could mean expanding weight, adding redundancies, or attempting progressed varieties.

7. Recovery and Rest:

- Permit muscles 48 hours of rest prior to focusing on a similar gathering.

- For recovery, prioritize getting enough sleep and eating well.

8. Maintain Consistency:

The key to getting results is being consistent.

- Aim for at least two or three sessions of strength training each week.

Strength preparing at home can be similarly basically as successful as in a rec center when drawn nearer with devotion and imagination. Tailor your daily practice to suit your inclinations, steadily increment power, and partake in the advantages of further developed strength, muscle tone, and in general prosperity.

Routines for Strength Training: Building Power and Flexibility

Integrating strength preparing into your wellness routine is vital for building muscle, improving digestion, and advancing generally practical wellness. Here is an example strength preparing routine for a full-body exercise:

Warm-Up:

- Cardio Warm-Up (5-10 minutes):

Bouncing jacks, high knees, or a light run to increment pulse.

- Dynamic Extending (5 minutes):

To get your muscles ready for movement, do arm circles, leg swings, and torso twists.

Full-Body Strength Exercise:

Each exercise should be performed in three sets of 12 to 15 repetitions. Change the weight and power based on your health.

1. Squats:

- Sit up straight with your feet shoulder-width apart.

While lowering your body into a sitting position, keep your knees over your lower legs.

- Press through heels to get back to the beginning position.

2. Push-Ups:

With your hands slightly wider than shoulder width, begin in the board position.

In the wake of bringing down your body in an orderly fashion from head to heels, propel yourself back up.

3. Rows of dolls stacked:

With your back straight and your hips turned, hold a free weight in each hand.

Pull the hand loads towards your chest, partner with your back muscles.

4. Lunges:

On one leg, move forward and lower your hips until your knees are twisted 90 degrees.

Switch legs and push back to the starting position.

5. Seat Plunges or Seats:

Place your hands beside your hips as you sit on the edge of a bench or chair and raise your body.

Press back up after lowering your body by bowing your elbows.

6. Deadlifts:

With an overhand grasp, hold a hand weight or free loads before you.

After lowering the weight with a hip pivot and maintaining a straight back, return to a standing position.

7. Plank:

 Keep your hands or forearms on the floor while you are in the plank position.

 By keeping a straight line from head to heels, you can work your center.

8. Curved Biceps:

 Hold a free weight in each hand while keeping your arms at your sides.

 Twist the loads toward your shoulders subsequent to dropping them back down.

9. Expansions of muscle in the rear arm:

With two hands, hold a free weight above you.

Fix your arms directly following turning at the elbows and putting the heap behind your head.

10. Changes in Russia:

Sit on the floor, lean back a little, and lift your legs off the ground.

Pivot your center so that each bend contacts the floor before you.

Cool Down:

- Five to ten minutes of static extension:
Hold each stretch for 15 to 30 seconds while you stretch the major muscle groups.

- Inhalation deeply (3-5 minutes):
Engage in practices that require you to inhale and exhale slowly and deeply.

Begin with a weight that expects you to invest some parcel of energy while as yet taking into consideration great structure, and steadily increment the power after some time. Attempt to play out every movement with fitting construction. If you are new to strength training or have any medical issues, speak with a health professional. Save a comparative regular practice for long stretch strength and wellbeing gains, yet transform it to suit your tendencies and the equipment you have accessible to you.

CHAPTER 6

Balanced Nutrition for Home Workouts: Fueling Your Fitness Journey

The best results from your home workouts come from more than just exercise; to support your energy levels, recovery, and overall well-being, you need to eat right. Here is a manual for keeping a fair eating regimen for your home gym routine daily schedule:

1. Hydration:

Relevance: Drink plenty of water to help your body absorb nutrients and support digestion.

A suggestion: Every day, drink at least 8 cups (64 ounces) of water. During intense workouts, increase intake.

2. Macronutrients:

Protein:

Significance: Fundamental for muscle fix and development.

Materials: Plant-based proteins like tofu and tempeh, lean poultry, fish, eggs, dairy, and legumes.

Carbohydrates:

Significance: primary source of energy for exercise.

Materials: Entire grains, natural products, vegetables, and vegetables.

Wholesome fats:

Significance: bolster overall health and supply lasting energy

Sources: olive oil, avocado, seeds, nuts, and fatty fish like salmon.

3. Nutrition for the Workout:

Timing: Eat a healthy meal two to three hours before you exercise.

Parts: Include some protein and some carbohydrates for energy.

Model: Banana and peanut butter on whole grain toast.

4. After-Workout Food:

Timing: Consume a feast or nibble inside 30-an hour in the wake of working out.

Elements: Carbohydrates to replenish glycogen stores and protein for muscle repair

Model: Greek yogurt topped with berries and nuts.

5. Example meals:

Breakfast:

Choice 1: Cereal with berries, chia seeds, and a spot of Greek yogurt.

Choice 2: Avocado, toast made of whole grain, scrambled eggs, and spinach

Lunch:

Choice 1: Mixed greens, quinoa, and a variety of vibrant vegetables make up this grilled chicken salad.

2nd Choice: Lentil and vegetable pan fried food with earthy colored rice.

Dinner:

Choice 1: steamed broccoli, sweet potato, and baked salmon.

2nd Choice: Chickpea curry with basmati rice and a side of blended vegetables.

Snacks:

Choice 1: Almonds and a handful of fresh fruit.

2nd Choice: Sliced strawberries and honey-drenched Greek yogurt.

6. Minerals and vitamins:

Relevance: Fundamental for generally well being and ideal body capability.

Sources: Make sure to include a wide range of colorful vegetables and fruits to get a wide range of vitamins and minerals.

7. When to Eat:

Consistency: In order to maintain a steady blood sugar level, aim for regular meal times.

Healthy Meals: Each meal should contain a combination of fats, carbohydrates, and protein.

8. Supplementation:

Thought: Before adding supplements, if necessary, consult a medical professional.

Normal Enhancements: Vitamin D, B nutrients, Omega-3 unsaturated fats, and protein powder in the event that dietary admission is lacking.

9. Reduce your intake of sugar-laden processed foods:

Objective: Support overall health and reduce inflammation.

Alternatives: Make use of natural sweeteners like honey or maple syrup and opt for whole, unprocessed foods.

10. Customization:

Specific Needs: Based on your preferences, dietary restrictions, and fitness objectives, modify your nutrition plan.

Try it out: Find what turns out best for your body and causes you to feel invigorated.

Portion Control and Mindful Eating: Nourishing Your Body with Awareness

Portion Control

Size The executives:

1. Utilize smaller dishes:

You can control how much you eat and give the impression of eating more by using smaller plates.

2. Think about Serving Sizes:

Learn about serving sizes to avoid revealing. The names of food sources can have strong associations.

3. fundamentally modify your diet:

Partition your plate into areas for vegetables, starches, and protein. In most cases, this ensures a healthy dinner.

4. Make an effort not to require additional snack immediately:

Prior to requiring a couple of moments, stand by some time. You should put money into your body if you want it to produce fruit.

5. Based on Evidence of Longing:

Listen to what your body is saying to you. Eat when you're full and stop when you're full.

6. Snacks for the event at the bar:

To prevent illegal use, quickly divide snacks into smaller, more sensible pieces.

7. Treats to share:

If you frequently dine out, split cakes can help you enjoy a sweet treat without overindulging.

Significance of portion control

Portion control is essential for a healthy lifestyle.

1. Holding calories under control:

Segments can be checked to limit calories. By eating in moderation, you can ensure that your body gets the energy it needs without being overloaded.

2. Controlling your weight:

It is essential to control the board's areas. By controlling how much you eat, you can keep a healthy weight and lower your risk of medical conditions linked to obesity.

3. Balance of supplements:

Upgrades can be produced at a reasonable cost with genuine piece control. By allowing you to eat up various food assortments, it ensures that you get a sufficient number of supplements, minerals, and macronutrients for your body.

4. Glucose Guideline:

Blood sugar levels are regulated by portion control. In order to improve metabolic health as a whole, consistent, well-balanced portions can help prevent spikes and crashes in blood sugar.

5. Stomach related Wellbeing:

Ideal part estimates support stomach related wellbeing. Overeating can put pressure on the digestive system, resulting in indigestion, discomfort, and other digestive issues.

6. Reduces Excessive Consumption:

More modest segments diminish the gamble of indulging. Keeping track of portion sizes supports weight loss or maintenance goals by preventing excessive calorie intake.

7. Instruction in Mindful Eating:

Segment control energizes careful dietary patterns. Monitoring segment sizes permits you to relish and partake in your food, advancing a better relationship with eating.

8. Boosts Your Energy Levels:

Consistent energy levels throughout the day are aided by portion control. Staying away from enormous, weighty feasts forestalls energy crashes and advances supported imperativeness.

9. Provides Variety:

A varied diet is encouraged by portion control. Partaking in various food sources in suitable sums guarantees you get an expansive scope of supplements from various food sources.

10. Mental Effect:

Segment control has mental advantages. It encourages a positive attitude toward living a healthy lifestyle by allowing you to indulge in a satisfying amount of food without feeling deprived.

11. Avoidance of Way of life Infections:

A lower risk of lifestyle diseases like diabetes, heart disease, and hypertension is linked to portion control. It improves overall well-being and health.

12. Reasonable Dietary patterns:

Eating in moderation fosters long-term eating habits. It's an approach to food consumption that can be sustained over time and is both realistic and manageable.

Basically, segment control is an essential part of keeping a fair and solid way of life. It supports overall well-being, weight management, and the prevention of various health issues by empowering individuals to make informed food choices.

Mindful Eating

1. Make contact with your teachers:

Take into account the variety, surfaces, and scents of your food. The eating experience is modified when you draw in your assets.

2. Eat without a care in the world:

Put away all screens and only focus on eating. This keeps you from indulging and assists you with perceiving when you're full.

3. Totally chew:

Take as much time as is needed and completely bite your food. This can assist with ingestion and movement toward your body when it is full.

4. Between Sizes for Nibbles:

Put your utensils down between meals. As a result of this, which maintains a speed that is more sluggish, you will actually want to see the value in each large piece.

5. In point of fact, examine the level of yearning:

Before and during the feast, assess your hunger. Do you like to eat at home or on a regular basis, or are you eager to try new restaurants?

6. Show your gratitude:

Take a moment to appreciate the value of the effort put into preparing your dinner. Your satisfaction in your food might be totally changed by this appreciation.

7. Be cautious when eating a lot:

Look for significant signs that could make you eat a ton. Find alternative means of coping with emotions that don't rely on food.

8. One aspect of mindfulness practice is:

Recognize the appropriate component. This mindfulness assists with forestalling nonsensical utilization.

9. Taste water in between snacks:

During your blowout, sip flavorful water to hydrate yourself. This makes it more straightforward to process and gives you an opportunity to stop.

10. Take in the entire picture:

Examine your body for signs of finish. Regardless of how much food you have left, quit eating when you are full.

11. Keep a food diary:

Monitor what, when, and how you eat. You will become more aware of your eating habits as a result of this training.

12. Recognize the Experiment:

Consider dinners as an encounter instead of an undertaking. Partake during the time spent sustaining your body.

By integrating segment control and careful eating rehearses, you can foster a better relationship with food. Not only do these routines help people lose weight, but they also make eating more mindful and enjoyable.

13. Consultation:

Advice from a professional: For specific guidance, think about speaking with a registered dietitian or nutritionist.

Including a variety of nutrient-dense foods, staying hydrated, and paying attention to your body's needs are all necessary components of a healthy diet. When it comes to your home workout routine and your nutrition, the key principles are consistency, variety, and moderation.

The Significance of Mindful Eating in a Healthy Lifestyle

1. Hunger and fullness awareness:

Careful eating cultivates an awareness of actual hunger and signs of fullness. This helps prevent overeating and encourages a more balanced approach to meals.

2. Enhanced Food Appreciation:

By eating mindfully, people can fully enjoy the flavors, textures, and aromas of their food. The general feasting experience is improved by this.

3. Expectations of Excessive Eating:

Cautious eating puts eating in light of sentiments, stress, or weakness. By empowering purposeful choices rather than rash ones, it energizes a better relationship with food.

4. Better absorption:

Processing is aided by being available and focused during dinner. Better processing and supplement intake are aided by eating food whole and at a slower pace.

5. Relationship with Body Signs:

People are able to distinguish genuine hunger from emotional or external triggers when they practice mindful eating because it creates a connection to internal cues.

6. The executives' weight:

Mindful eating is associated with better weight management. Being delicate to the body's signs helps individuals with chasing after informed choices about portion sizes and food decisions.

7. Weight Loss Prevention:

Careful eating lessens the probability of gorging by empowering a cognizant and deliberate way to deal with feasts. Weight loss and weight maintenance goals may benefit from this.

8. Changes automatic eating patterns:

Mindful eating breaks eating habits that are automatic or habitual. It prompts people to pursue intentional decisions, prompting a more adjusted and wellbeing cognizant eating regimen.

9. Positive Emotional State:

Taking part in careful eating upholds close to home prosperity. It fosters a healthier relationship with one's body and self-image, fostering a positive and non-judgmental attitude toward food.

10. Anticipation of Voraciously consuming food:

It has been demonstrated that mindful eating strategies work to prevent binge eating episodes. People can avoid overindulging in food in a short amount of time by being present during meals.

11. Connection Between the Mind and the Body:

The mind-body connection is strengthened by mindful eating. Focusing on what food means for the body elevates a comprehensive way to deal with wellbeing and prosperity.

12. Enhanced Food Satisfaction:

By relishing each nibble and focusing on the eating experience, people can get more noteworthy fulfillment from their dinners, lessening the longing for pointless nibbling.

13. Expanded Appreciation for Food:

Being careful encourages appreciation for the food we have. It helps people appreciate the work that goes into producing food and the nourishment it provides.

Generally, careful eating is a strong practice that goes past simple sustenance. It includes a comprehensive way to deal with food, cultivating a positive relationship with eating, advancing close to home prosperity, and adding to long haul wellbeing and fulfillment.

CHAPTER 7

Staying Motivated: A Guide to Consistency in Your Fitness Journey

Understanding Motivation:

Establish Your "Why":

Obviously express why you set out on your wellness process. Whether it's superior wellbeing, expanded energy, or a particular objective, realizing your motivation upgrades inspiration.

Put forth Sensible Objectives:

Lay out reachable and quantifiable objectives. Break them down into smaller anniversaries to mark the progress.

Imagining Success:

Visualize the good things that will come from achieving your fitness goals. Perception can build up your responsibility and keep you centered.

Embrace Assortment:

Make sure your workouts are varied and fun. Attempting new activities or exercises forestalls repetitiveness and adds fervor to your daily schedule.

Increasing Consistency:

Establish a routine:

Lay out a predictable exercise plan. A normal coordinate practice into your everyday existence, making it a non-debatable piece of your day.

Responsibility Accomplices:

Tell a friend or family member your fitness goals. Having somebody to impart accomplishments and difficulties to adds a social part to your excursion.

Keep tabs on Your Development:

Record your achievements. Routinely survey how far you've come to see the value in your accomplishments and remain persuaded.

Flexibility is crucial:

Approach with adaptability. Life might introduce unforeseen difficulties, yet having an adaptable mentality permits you to change your arrangements without wrecking your advancement.

Overcoming Obstacles:

Expect Misfortunes:

Accept that failures are an inevitable part of any journey. Take what you've learned from them, tweak your strategy, and move on.

Recognize Small Successes:

Recognize and rejoice in even the smallest accomplishments. Your success is influenced by every small step you take.

Talking well of oneself:

Replace negative thoughts with affirmations that are positive. Empower yourself and spotlight your capacities instead of seeing restrictions.

Track down Euphoria Simultaneously:

Find the aspects of your exercise routine that make you happy. Whether it's a most loved practice or the sensation of achievement after an exercise, develop delight in the excursion.

Supporting Inspiration Long haul:

Consolidate Prizes:

Create a system for rewarding achievement of milestones. Give yourself a treat that will make you feel good about your efforts to get in shape.

Keep up-to-date and inspired:

To remain enthusiastic and motivated about your fitness journey, read about fitness success stories, follow inspirational figures on social media, or investigate new workout trends.

Join People group:

Associate with similar people. On the web or nearby wellness networks offer help, consolation, and a feeling of having a place.

Re-examine and re-frame:

Make any necessary adjustments to your goals at regular intervals. Embrace the valuable chance to develop and develop alongside your wellness process.

Give Self-Care Priority:

Recognize the significance of recuperation and rest. Dealing with your psychological and actual prosperity adds to supported inspiration.

Consider Your "Why":

Review your initial motivations for starting your fitness journey on a regular basis. Your commitment is renewed when you reconnect with your motivations.

Keep in mind, remaining spurred is a unique cycle that requires exertion and self-reflection. You can cultivate long-term dedication to your fitness goals by comprehending your motivations, developing consistency, overcoming obstacles, and incorporating sustainable practices.

The Significance of Motivation in Achieving Goals

1. Starts the Action:

People are motivated to take action because it is the driving force behind their actions. The spark that sets off the journey toward achieving objectives is this.

2. Prevents Effort:

Despite challenges, inspiration goes about as a supporting element. It enables individuals to persevere and remain committed to their goals despite obstacles.

3. Conquers Snags:

The resilience necessary to overcome obstacles is provided by motivation. It encourages people to see challenges not as insurmountable obstacles but rather as opportunities for growth.

4. Clarity of Objective:

Goals become crystal clear when motivated. It provides individuals with a clear path for their efforts and helps them define what they want to accomplish and why.

5. Improves Focus:

Inspiration homes concentrate on explicit undertakings and goals. It limits interruptions and keeps people on target toward their ideal results.

6. Helps Certainty:

Self-confidence rises when one is motivated to succeed and make progress. The belief that goals are attainable is bolstered by achieving even the smallest milestones.

7. Encourages Originality:

Motivation encourages inventive thinking and creativity. It inspires individuals to investigate novel strategies and solutions for overcoming obstacles.

8. Enhances Efficiency:

Motivated people typically perform at a higher level. The desire to achieve objectives frequently results in increased effort, dedication, and improved performance as a whole.

9. Cultivates Positive Attitude:

A positive outlook is cultivated through motivation. It fosters resilience and mental well-being by assisting individuals to maintain an optimistic outlook even in the face of setbacks.

10. Facilitates Making Decisions:

Motivation helps people make decisions. People are more likely to make decisions that are in line with their goals, values, and long-term vision when they are motivated.

11. Boosts Personal Development:

Motivation is a driving force behind personal development. It encourages people to step outside of their comfort zones, accept challenges, and continue to grow.

12. Fortifies Responsibility:

Commitment to goals is boosted by motivation. People who are persuaded are bound to remain devoted and finish their arrangements.

13. Develops Flexibility:

Resilience is aided by motivation. It urges people to return from mishaps, gain from disappointments, and endure chasing after their yearnings.

14. Makes a Positive Criticism Circle:

A positive feedback loop is created when success is driven by motivation. When goals are met, people are more motivated to set and pursue new goals.

15. Upgrades Profound Prosperity:

Inspiration is connected to profound prosperity. Chasing after significant objectives gives a feeling of motivation and satisfaction, emphatically influencing generally emotional well-being.

16. Encourages Good Habits:

When it comes to developing and sustaining healthy habits, motivation is of the utmost importance. It drives people to take on ways of behaving that line up with their prosperity objectives.

17. Increases momentum:

Inspiration makes energy. Little victories expand on one another, producing a feeling of progress and moving people forward on their excursion.

18. Cultivates a Compensating Excursion:

In the end, motivation makes achieving goals a fulfilling journey. It imbues reason and energy into activities, making the whole interaction satisfying and significant.

In conclusion, motivation is a dynamic force that encourages people to act, overcome obstacles, and realize their goals. It is the driving force behind persistent effort, achievement of objectives, and personal development.

Crafting Your Home Workout Schedule: A Blueprint for Success

1. Examine your accessibility:

Consistently complete the available movement times. Plan how you'll finish your work and think about your own preferences and commitments to your family.

2. Important consistency is:

Choose a regular time to exercise. Making exercise a priority in your daily life and sticking to a schedule becomes easier as a result of this.

3. Morning Activator:

Advantages: Once more, assist your digestion.

Support levels of energy over the course of the day.

An example: 7:00 AM - 8:00 AM

4. Get a quick break in the early evening:

Advantages:

Separate the regular workday.

Give your body and mind some time off.

Model: 12:30 PM - 1:00 PM

5. An Improvement for the Following Day:

Benefits:

Get out of your morning hangover.

Enhance productivity and focus.

An occurrence: 4:30 PM - 5:30 PM

6. This was what the destroyer did in the evening:

Advantages:

Let go of the stress of the day.

Release any tension that has developed.

A logical analysis: 7:00 PM - 8:00 PM

7. Rival at the week's end:

Advantages: An opportunity to move around outside; - a restriction on doing more activities.Model: Saturday or Sunday, 9:00 AM - 10:30 AM

8. Choose your working days:

A concept:

Attempt to practice some place near three and five days out of each and every week.

Exercises that consolidate collaboration, cardio, and adaptability

Significance:

Give your body time to heal.

Lessening the likelihood of harm and avoidable burnout.

Some heading: Plan a couple of days off each week.

10. Give yourself a break:

Consider:

Rehearses that are more confined and more associated with can be helpful.

You can design longer meetings for a really long time when you have additional time.

11. Be flexible and versatile:

The Approach:

Schedules can shift as life happens.

Think about other options for busy days.

12. Alter Your Daily Routine:

Benefits:

Stop levels and weaknesses.

Incorporate a wide range of muscle groups.

Model:

Monday: Tuesday: Strength organizing: Cardio day is on Wednesday: Yoga

Thursday: Practice on Friday: Versatility and Convenience in HIIT 13. Set up alerts or updates:

Tip:

To kick you off on your work-out daily practice, remember alerts or updates for your timetable.

Approach it as a crucial appointment.

14. Include a cool-down as well as a warm-up:

A change:

Give yourself time to warm up and relax before the workout.

- Increase adaptability, avoid injury, and speed up recovery 15 Get your arrangement on paper:

- Benefit:

Make use of apps or an exercise log to monitor your progress.

- Appreciate achievements and adapt your schedule to the situation.

16. Examine Achievements:

- Appreciation:

Consider your endeavors and accomplishments.

- Give monetary impetuses to accomplishing explicit wellbeing objectives.

17. Stay flexible:

- Flexibility:

You shouldn't be ashamed of changing your schedule because needs can change in major strength areas for a.

Consider the fact that your home workout routine should be tailored to your preferences and lifestyle. The emphasis is on adaptability and consistency, so feel free to look around until you find a routine that inspires and empowers you.

CHAPTER 8

Overcoming Challenges

Embracing Your Human Journey Home workouts can help you fit exercise into your busy schedule while saving money on gym memberships. In any case, there are a few difficulties that can make it hard to stay with a home exercise routine daily schedule. Here are a few ways to conquer these difficulties:

1. Recognize the Obstacle:

- Recognize and accept the obstacle in front of you. The first step toward overcoming it is acknowledging it.

2. Take it apart:

- Partition the test into more modest, more sensible undertakings. Taking the process one step at a time makes it less overwhelming.

3. Seek Assistance:

- Go ahead and out to companions, family, or associates. Sharing your difficulty can help you gain new perspectives and emotional support.

4. Learn and Adjust:

- See difficulties as opportunities for development. Take into account the lessons they teach you and modify your strategy accordingly.

5. Set Practical Assumptions:

- Be sensible about what you can accomplish. Putting forth attainable objectives forestalls superfluous pressure and frustration.

6. Self-Care and mindfulness:

- To remain present and control stress, practice mindfulness. Be understanding of yourself; Obstacles are a part of life for everyone.

7. Recognize Small Successes:

- Recognize and praise each little triumph. Your overall progress is aided by every, no matter how insignificant, step you take forward.

8. Accept Change:

- Recognize that life is always changing. Embracing it, in any event, while testing, makes the way for additional opportunities.

9. Gain from Difficulties:

- Rather than harping on mishaps, use them as any open door to learn and move along. Flexibility is worked through beating snags.

10. Affirmations that are Good:

- Replace negative thoughts with affirmations that are positive. Remind yourself of your abilities and strengths.

11. Focus on Taking care of oneself:

- Take care of your mental and physical health. Taking care of oneself gives the strength expected to deal with difficulties directly.

12. Make a Strategy:

- Come up with a plan to deal with the problem. A sense of control and direction are provided by having a plan in place.

13. Be Proud of Your Humanity:

- Recognize that being human necessitates overcoming obstacles. It's a common encounter, and looking for help is an indication of solidarity, not shortcoming.

14. Foster Strength:

A person's resilience grows stronger with each challenge. Consider challenges as opportunities to strengthen your resilience.

15. Concentrate on Options:

- Instead of dwelling on the issue, concentrate on possible solutions. An answer situated mentality engages you to make a move.

16. Be able to say no:

- Saying no when necessary is OK. To effectively manage challenges and maintain equilibrium, setting boundaries is essential.

17. Maintain Perspective:

- Keep a more extensive viewpoint. Keeping an eye on the bigger picture can be motivating, and challenges typically last only a short time.

18. Observe Your Excursion:

- Ponder how far you've come. Your ability to overcome any obstacle is evidence of your strength and resilience.

Keep in mind, challenges are a fundamental piece of the human experience. You will not only overcome the immediate obstacle but also develop as a person by approaching them with a positive attitude, seeking support, and learning from the process.

Dealing with Plateaus

Home activities and noticing levels are indistinguishable on any movement plan. Giving up can sometimes be both frustrating and tempting. However, there are two ways to complete a level:

Investigate and learn about:
Make a stride back and check out at the circumstance according to an objective viewpoint. Keep in mind that levels are an important part of every outing.

Reconsider Your Approach:
Break down your tendency for conventional movement and diet. Find out which parts need to be changed or could have been compromised. You doubtlessly notice no movements in your body if you've been doing things

the same way for quite a while. Consider integrating new exercises or practicing at a higher power.

Focus on how you make it. You can keep yourself motivated and see how far you have come by tracking your workouts and progress. To keep tabs on your development, you can utilize an assortment of applications and sites.

Choose a companion to move with. Working out with a partner can help you stay accountable and motivated. Online or in your own space, you can also find practice colleagues.

Reward yourself: At the point when you achieve something, reward yourself with something you esteem. You'll stay motivated and have more fun working out as a result.

Managing Stress and Emotional Eating

Keeping a good dieting and work-out routine can be troublesome while managing pressure and essential eating issues. Focusing on the board and eating at home: Try the following if you notice that you are unable to control your stress or that you eat more when you are stressed:

Find out what triggers you; What regularly induces anxiety in you? Once you have identified your triggers, you can begin devising strategies for either avoiding them or managing them.

Find healthy approaches to stress management: The pioneers made pressure mitigating techniques that included yoga, reflection, exercise, and contributing energy with friends and family.

Assume responsibility for your nourishment: Pay attention to signs of longing and eat when you're really hungry. Eat possibly when you are powerless, drained, or focused.

Keep unhealthy food sources out of the house. You are more likely to avoid eating unhealthy foods if there is no food in the house.

Find a group that welcomes new concepts: Discuss your preferences with a friend, family member, or organized professional. Talking to someone can make you feel like you've accomplished a lot and help you focus on your goals.

Recollect that no two people are something basically the same, and the methodologies that are convincing for one individual most likely will not be suitable for another. Give two or three options a shot and see which one proves to be the most challenging for you.

The Negative Effects of Insignificant Eating on the Execution of Home Confinement:

1. Being extremely close and continuing to hang out there due to stress or hopeless assumptions can lead to shameful food choices. When you eat bad food, you might feel sluggish and need more energy, making it hard to get started on family chores.

2. Genuine Wellbeing Objectives:

   When eating, individuals typically consume food sources that are low in supplements and high in calories. When diverged from the work put into practices at home, standard indulgences can hinder progress toward wellbeing objectives and add to weight gain.

3. An improvement to the flaw:

   Changes in glucose levels could result from express wellsprings of comfort food that are associated with home cooking. Because this can make you feel more drained, it might be helpful to try to maintain a similar level of force and consistency for practical home activities.

4. Nonattendance of Motivation:

    A debilitating circle of possibility and shame can be worked up by particularly close eating, which makes a problematic mental difference. Keeping up a standard gym routine everyday practice at home might be more troublesome given this weight.

5. Hazard of Overtraining:

    The risk of overtraining can rise when a single responds to feelings by going out into the unknown and adhering to established dietary guidelines. Overtraining can make you really tired, make it take more effort to complete tasks, and increase your risk of injury.

6. Recovery in darkness:

    Analyzing bad food as part of profound eating may be included. The body's ability to recover from exercise can be hindered by disruption, resulting in recognized aggravation and delayed progress.

7. twisted self-insight:

    When combined with skeptical sentiments, eating near and dear can fuel twisted self-revelation. This changed information could totally influence your affirmation and demeanor toward your undertakings to move into your home.

8. Hot Ways Of eating:

    Eating in close proximity occasionally disrupts conventional eating patterns. If you eat frequently or frequently, your body may not be able to properly refuel and recover from activities at home.

9. Heightened feelings of tension:

    Eating in moderation can exacerbate stress. Foods that make people feel good may help for a short time, but over time, they may make people feel more restless, which is bad for their mental and physical health.

10. Non Appearance of drive to work out:

    When you indulge, it can be difficult to complete tasks at home. The advantages of dynamic work might lessen assuming that action is related with hasty or despicable family eating.

11. Demand from Local Overflow:

    The trouble of friends and family is every now and again connected to indulging. Because of the impact on mental flourishing, which can show up in various ways, totally participating in home activities with a creating perspective may be basically more pursuing for you.

12. Unusual behavior on one's part:

Engaging in something can demonstrate bad behavior. By accepting that the essential reasons individuals eat continue as before, we could have an interminable rundown of doubtful contemplations and ways of cheating.

To keep a positive and necessary home exercise routine, fundamental eating plans must be examined and addressed. By developing solid areas for an association between your sentiments and food, you can work on both your psychological and actual wellbeing. As a result, the exercises you do at home will actually want to contribute to your overall health goals.

CHAPTER 9

Celebrating your success

1. Commending your triumphs, both of all shapes and sizes, is a significant piece of having a decent outlook on yourself and remaining persuaded to accomplish your objectives. Here are a few hints on the most proficient method to praise your victories:

2. Carve out opportunity to see the value in your achievements. Try not to simply forget about them as not a problem. Pause for a minute to consider what you've accomplished and how hard you attempted to arrive.

3. Share your triumphs with others. Tell your companions, family, and collaborators about your achievements. They will be glad for yourself and it will support your certainty.

4. Indulge yourself with something you appreciate. Get yourself another outfit, get a back rub, or go out for a decent supper. This is an approach to

compensating yourself for your diligent effort and supporting a positive way of behaving.

5. Put away the opportunity to celebrate. Assuming you're feeling overpowered, don't attempt to celebrate everything simultaneously. Put away a period every week or month to consider your achievements and praise your triumphs.

6. Feel free to commend your little victories. Indeed, even little victories merit celebration. They are an update that you are gaining ground and that you are fit for accomplishing your objectives.

7. Utilize your triumphs as inspiration to continue to push ahead. At the point when you commend your victories, it will help you to remember how far you've come and propel you to continue to pursue your objectives.

8. Practice it regularly to praise your victories. The more you commend your triumphs, the more sure you will become and the more probable you are to accomplish your objectives.

9. Figure out how to praise that function for you. There is no correct method for celebrating. Find a way that causes you to feel significantly better and that squeezes into your way of life.

10. Try not to contrast your triumphs with others. Everybody's process is unique. Commend your own victories and don't stress over the things others are doing.

11. Celebrate your triumphs constantly. Regardless of how enormous or little, your victories merit celebrating. So carve out opportunity to see the value in your achievements and partake in the sensation of accomplishment.

Here are some ideas for how to celebrate your successes:

Go on an outing. This could be an end of the week escape or a long excursion.

Get yourself something you've been needing. This could be another outfit, a piece of gems, or a device.

Go out to eat at a pleasant café. This is an extraordinary method for treating yourself and commend your achievement.

Host a get-together with your loved ones. This is a pleasant method for imparting your prosperity to individuals you care about.

Accomplish something you appreciate. This could be perusing, going for a stroll, or investing energy with your friends and family.

Give to your #1 cause. This is an incredible method for rewarding your local area and warm hearted about yourself.

Record your triumphs in a diary. This is an incredible method for keeping tabs on your development and consider your achievements.

Make a dream board. This is an incredible method for picturing your objectives and keep tabs on your development.

Share your triumphs via web-based entertainment. This is an incredible method for interfacing with others and offer your positive encounters.

Regardless of how you decide to celebrate, ensure it is something that you appreciate and that helps you have a positive outlook on yourself. Commending your triumphs is an approach to recognizing your persistent effort and supporting positive way of behaving. It is likewise an approach to inspiring yourself to continue to push ahead and accomplish your objectives.

At the point when you praise your victories, you are making an impression on yourself that you are fit for accomplishing extraordinary things. This can support your certainty and assist you with making significantly more progress from here on out. So find opportunity to praise your triumphs, of all shapes and sizes. You merit it!

CONCLUSION

As we arrive at the summit of this book, it's a consummation as well as a festival of your excursion towards a better and more dynamic life. All through these pages, we've investigated the fundamental components of setting and accomplishing wellbeing and health objectives in the solace of your home.

From characterizing your ideal body and laying out reasonable objectives to understanding the meaning of careful eating and part control, you've acquired significant bits of knowledge into developing an economical and adjusted way of life. The excursion doesn't end here; it changes into a deep rooted obligation to your prosperity.

By perceiving the significance of inspiration, you've outfitted the ability to defeat difficulties, get through levels, and praise your victories, both of all shapes and sizes. Keep in mind, this isn't simply a book; an aide engages you to assume responsibility for your wellbeing and embrace a positive and careful way to deal with living.

As you push ahead, keep on paying attention to your body, put forth new objectives, and adjust your techniques. Embrace the standards of careful living, praise each step of your excursion, and perceive that your obligation to a better way of life is a gift to yourself.

Your way to health is exceptionally yours, and this book fills in as a compass, giving direction and consolation. The parts you've investigated are not simply words on pages; they are venturing stones, making ready for a better, more joyful, and more satisfied you.

May your process be loaded up with self-revelation, strength, and the delight of accomplishing the wellbeing and health you merit. Here's to the following part in your lively and engaged life!

APPENDIX

SIMPLE NUTRITIOUS RECIPES

Breakfast:

1. Spinach and Egg Scramble with Raspberries

This speedy egg scramble with generous bread is one of the most mind-blowing morning meals for weight loss. Whole-grain toast and spinach, as well as protein-packed eggs and superfood raspberries, make up this dish. The protein and fiber give you a filling breakfast that keeps you going all morning.

Time for preparation: 10 minutes in total: 10 mins

Servings: 1

Fixings

Yield: Serving Size: 1 serving

1 teaspoon canola oil

1 ½ cups child spinach (1 1/2 ounces)

2 huge eggs, delicately beaten

Touch of legitimate salt

Touch of ground pepper

1 cut entire grain bread, toasted

½ cup new raspberries

Instructions

Heat oil in a little nonstick skillet over medium-high intensity. Cook spinach for one to two minutes, stirring frequently, until wilted. Move the spinach to a plate. Place the pan over medium heat, clean it, and add the eggs. Cook, mixing a few times to guarantee in any event, cooking, until recently set, 1 to 2 minutes. Add the salt and pepper, spinach, and stir. Toast and raspberries can be added to the scrambled eggs.

2. Berry-Almond Smoothie Bowl A little frozen banana gives this filling smoothie bowl a creamy texture.

Planning Time: 10 minutes

in total: 10 minutes

Serves: 1

Yield: 1 serving

Fixings:

2/3 cup frozen raspberries

1/12 cup frozen sliced banana

1/12 cup plain unsweetened almond milk

5 tablespoons sliced almonds, divided

1/4 teaspoon ground cinnamon

1/8 teaspoon ground cardamom

1/8 teaspoon vanilla extract

1/4 cup blueberries

1 tablespoon unsweetened coconut flakes

Instructions

In a blender, blend the raspberries, banana, almond milk, cinnamon, cardamom, and vanilla until very smooth.

Empty the smoothie into a bowl and top with blueberries, the leftover 2 tablespoons of almonds and coconut.

3. **Smoothie Bowl with Raspberry, Peach, and Mango**

This nutritious smoothie recipe is an introduction to the smoothie bowl craze. Utilize anything that is an organic product, nuts and seeds you like best to make it your own. Make certain to involve frozen natural product in Sync 1 to yield a smooth, cold base for the garnishes.

Time to Cook: 10 mins

All out Time: 10 minutes

Serves: 1

Yield: 1 serving

Fixings

1 cup frozen mango lumps

¾ cup nonfat plain Greek yogurt

¼ cup diminished fat milk

1 teaspoon vanilla concentrate

¼ ready peach, cut

⅓ cup raspberries

1 tablespoon cut almonds, toasted whenever wanted

1 tablespoon unsweetened coconut chips, toasted whenever wanted

1 teaspoon chia seeds

Instructions

Consolidate mango, yogurt, milk and vanilla in a blender. Blend till smooth.

To taste, top the smoothie with almonds, peach slices, raspberries, coconut, and chia seeds.

4. Avocado & Kale Omelet

For a filling, high-protein breakfast, make this omelet with kale and avocado. In this healthy omelet recipe, the fiber-rich kale will keep you fuller for a longer period of time.

Prep Time: 10 mins

Total Time: 10 mins

Servings: 1

Yield: 1 serving

Ingredients

2 large eggs

1 teaspoon low-fat milk

Pinch of salt

2 teaspoons extra-virgin olive oil, divided

1 cup chopped kale

1 tablespoon lime juice

1 tablespoon chopped fresh cilantro

1 teaspoon unsalted sunflower seeds

Pinch of crushed red pepper

Pinch of salt

¼ avocado, sliced

Directions

In a little bowl, beat the eggs, milk, and salt together. In a small nonstick skillet, heat 1 teaspoon of oil over medium heat. Cook for one to two minutes, then add the egg mixture and cook until the bottom is set but the center is still a little runny. Flip the omelet over and cook until set, around 30 seconds more. Place on a plate.

Throw kale with the excess 1 teaspoon oil, lime juice, cilantro, sunflower seeds, crushed red pepper and a touch of salt. Avocado and the kale salad should be added to the omelet.

5. Oatmeal-Almond Protein Pancakes

The amount of liquid in this protein pancake recipe may need to be reduced depending on the protein powder you use. Whey-protein hotcakes need less fluid than those made with soy, hemp or pea protein. With yogurt and a homemade fruit sauce made from warmed frozen berries and a pinch of sugar, serve.

Cook Time: 30 mins

Additional Time: 15 mins

Total Time: 45 mins

Servings: 4

Yield: 4 servings

Ingredients

½ cup unflavored protein powder

½ cup almond meal

½ cup oat flour (see Tip)

1 tablespoon sugar

1 teaspoon ground cinnamon

1 teaspoon baking powder

¼ teaspoon baking soda

¼ teaspoon salt

2 large eggs

¾ cup buttermilk

2 tablespoons canola oil

2 teaspoons vanilla extract

In a blender, combine the protein powder, oat flour, almond meal, sugar, cinnamon, baking powder, baking soda, and salt; beat until completely blended. Oil, vanilla, the eggs (reduce to 1/2 cup if using whey protein), and buttermilk pulse, stopping whenever necessary to scrape down the sides, until combined. Allow to sit for 15 minutes.

Cover a huge nonstick skillet or frying pan with cooking splash; heat over medium-high intensity.

Using1/4 mug batter per hotcake, make roughly three flapjacks at a time; Set the temperature to medium. Cook for 1 to 3 twinkles or until the edges are dry. Flip and cook until brilliant brown on the contrary side, 1 to 3 twinkles more. Using further cuisine spray and conforming the heat as necessary, carry out the process with the remaining batter. Serve warm.

Tips

Oat flour is produced using finely processed entire oats. Whole grains and dietary fiber are abundant in it. Attempt it instead of a part of other flour in recipes like hotcakes, fast breads and biscuits. Look for it near gluten-free flours or in other whole-grain flours. Alternatively, you can make your own by grinding traditional rolled oats in a blender or food processor until they resemble flour.

6. Muffin-Tin Quiches with Smoked Cheddar & Potato

This recipe for a mini quiche is delicious and filling thanks to the potatoes, cheese, and greens. You can quickly prepare breakfast for the rest of the week by baking a batch over the weekend.

Time for preparation: 30 minutes

More time: 30 mins

Absolute Time: 1 hour

Serving Size: 6

Yield: 6 servings

Ingredients

2 tablespoons extra-virgin olive oil

1 ½ cups finely diced red-skinned potatoes

1 cup diced red onion

¾ teaspoon salt, divided

8 large eggs

1 cup shredded smoked Cheddar cheese

½ cup low-fat milk

½ teaspoon ground black pepper

1 ½ cups chopped fresh spinach

Instructions

Spray a 12-cup muffin pan with cooking spray and heat the oven to 325 degrees F.

In a large skillet, heat the oil to medium-high heat. Add potatoes, onion and 1/4 teaspoon salt and cook, mixing, until the potatoes are simply cooked through, around 5 minutes. Eliminate intensity and let cool for 5 minutes.

In a large bowl, combine the eggs, cheese, milk, pepper, and the remaining 1/2 teaspoon of salt. Mix in spinach and the potato combination. Split the quiche combination between the pre-arranged biscuit cups.

Prepare until firm to the touch, around 25 minutes. Before removing from the tin, let it stand for five minutes.

Tip

To make ahead: Wrap each one in plastic and store in the refrigerator for up to three days or freeze for up to one month. To warm, eliminate plastic, enclose it with a paper towel and microwave on High for 30 to 60 seconds.

7. Baby Kale Breakfast Salad with Bacon & Egg

Salad for breakfast? Oh yes! Get your day going right with this sound breakfast recipe. With your first meal of the day, you can get half of your daily vegetable intake from a bowl of healthy greens like baby kale.

Cook Time: 15 mins

Total Time: 15 mins

Servings: 1

Yield: 1 serving

Ingredients

1 teaspoon minced garlic

Pinch of salt

1 tablespoon extra-virgin olive oil

2 teaspoons red-wine vinegar

Pinch of ground pepper

3 cups lightly packed baby kale

1 piece cooked bacon, chopped

1 fried or poached large egg

Instructions:

Make a paste by combining the salt and garlic with the side of a chef's knife or a fork. In a medium bowl, combine the oil, vinegar, pepper, and garlic paste. Include kale throw to cover. Serve the kale salad finished off with bacon and egg.

Lunch

1. Macaroni Salad with Creamy Avocado Dressing

Give exemplary pasta salad a fresher, more tasty twist. Avocado replaces some of the mayonnaise in this quick pasta dish, making it even creamier. This healthy pasta salad is made with elbow macaroni made from whole wheat and fresh vegetables. You'll be making it all summer long.

Time Active: 25 mins

Complete Time: 25 mins

Servings: 12

Yield: 12 servings

Ingredients

8 ounces entire wheat elbow macaroni (around 2 cups)

1 cup cleaved red chime pepper

½ cup meagerly cut celery

2 scallions, cleaved

2 tablespoons cleaved new parsley or cilantro

1 ready medium avocado

¼ cup mayonnaise

2 tablespoons rice vinegar

¾ teaspoon salt

½ teaspoon dried minced garlic

¼ teaspoon ground pepper

Directions

Cook macaroni in a huge pot of bubbling water as per bundle headings. Rinse with ice water after draining; again drain Move into a large bowl. Scallions, bell pepper, celery, and parsley (or cilantro) should be added.

Take the avocado in half, remove the pit, and put the flesh in a small food processor. Add mayonnaise, vinegar, salt, pepper, and dried garlic. Process until smooth. Combine the macaroni salad and avocado dressing in a large bowl and stir until well coated.

Note: To make ahead; Refrigerate for as long as 1 day.

2. Bacon-Lettuce-Avocado-Tomato Sandwiches

In this solid BLT recipe, we utilize a velvety avocado spread enhanced with garlic and basil, and add sprouts. Search for grown wheat bread in the frozen area or with other specialty breads at your supermarket.

Time to Cook: 25 mins

Complete Time: 25 mins

Servings: 4

Yield: 4 servings

Ingredients

8 cuts place cut bacon, split

1 ready medium avocado

2 tablespoons cleaved new basil

1 tablespoon mayonnaise

½ teaspoon finely ground or minced garlic

¼ teaspoon salt

¼ teaspoon ground pepper

8 cuts grew wheat bread

1 medium tomato, cut into 8 cuts

4 romaine leaves

1 cup horse feed sprouts

Directions

In a large skillet, cook the bacon for 5 to 10 minutes on medium heat until crisp. Transfer to a paper towel-lined plate.

Squash the avocado in a medium bowl while you wait. Garlic, basil, mayonnaise, salt, and pepper are all added. Cook bread.

On four pieces of toast, spread about 2 tablespoons of the avocado mixture. Each with the remaining toast, two tomato slices, one lettuce leaf, one-fourth of a cup of sprouts, and four pieces of bacon.

3. Spinach and Mushroom Quiche

This solid vegan quiche recipe is pretty much basic. Without the fussy crust, it tastes like quiche! Sweet wild mushrooms and savory Gruyère cheese fill it. Serve it with a light salad for lunch or for breakfast or brunch.

Time Active: 25 mins

Complete Time: 1 hr 5 mins

Servings: 6

Yield: 1 quiche

Ingredients

2 tablespoons extra-virgin olive oil

8 ounces sliced fresh mixed wild mushrooms such as cremini, shiitake, button and/or oyster mushrooms

1 ½ cups thinly sliced sweet onion (If you don't have a sweet onion, you can use a white onion or yellow onion as a substitute in this recipe because they taste milder when cooked.)

1 tablespoon thinly sliced garlic

5 ounces fresh baby spinach (about 8 cups), coarsely chopped (frozen spinach can be used as substitute)

6 large eggs

¼ cup whole milk

¼ cup half-and-half

1 tablespoon Dijon mustard

1 tablespoon fresh thyme leaves, plus more for garnish

¼ teaspoon salt

¼ teaspoon ground pepper

1 ½ cups shredded Gruyère cheese (Swiss, Gouda or Cheddar can be used as substitute)

Instructions:

Shower a pie dish that is 9 creeps in width with cooking splash and preheat the broiler to 375 degrees Fahrenheit.

Heat the oil to medium-high heat in a large nonstick skillet; Swirl the pan to coat it. Include the mushrooms and cook for about 8 minutes, occasionally blending, until they are caramelized and delicate. Integrate garlic and onion; cook, mixing as frequently as possible, for approximately 5 minutes until loose and fragile. Add spinach; cook for one to two minutes, tossing frequently, until wilted. Turn off the heat.

In a medium bowl, join the eggs, milk, cream, mustard, thyme, salt, and pepper. Incorporate the cheddar and the combination of mushrooms. Split between the pre-arranged pie dishes. Heat for about 30 minutes until set and splendid brown. Give the speech ten minutes; slice. Present with thyme as an upgrade.

Note:

Up to five days in advance, cover and refrigerate spinach and mushroom quiche. Cover and microwave or warm the entire quiche in the microwave by the slice at 350°F for 30 to 45 minutes.

4.   Loaded Cucumber & Avocado Sandwich

Crispy cucumbers and creamy avocado fill this loaded cucumber-and-avocado sandwich. Ricotta cheddar blended in with extra-sharp Cheddar adds flavor while cut red peppers offer a sprinkle of variety.

Active Time: 10 mins
Total Time: 10 mins
Servings: 1

Ingredients

3 tablespoons shredded extra-sharp Cheddar cheese

2 tablespoons ricotta cheese

4 teaspoons finely sliced chives

2 teaspoons lemon juice

Ground pepper to taste

2 slices whole-wheat sandwich bread, lightly toasted

⅓ cup thinly sliced cucumber

¼ cup thinly sliced red bell pepper

⅓ avocado, sliced

instructions

Mix Cheddar, ricotta, chives, lemon squeeze, salt and pepper together in a little bowl. Spread around 50% of the blend on each cut of toast. Layer one cut with cucumber, pepper and avocado, then top with the other cut, spread-side down.

5. Bowl of Cauliflower Rice and Chipotle Chicken Burrito

This simple to-make and feast prep burrito bowl is far better than takeout! This protein-packed, incredibly flavorful dish, in which cauliflower rice takes the place of cilantro-lime rice, will never make you miss the carbs. We love this with chicken, but shrimp would also be great.

Prep Time: 35 mins

Additional Time: 10 mins

Total Time: 45 mins

Servings: 4

Yield: 4 bowls

Ingredients

4 cups cauliflower florets

3 tablespoons extra-virgin olive oil, divided

½ teaspoon salt, divided

1 pound skinless, boneless chicken breasts

1 tablespoon finely chopped chipotle peppers in adobo sauce

½ teaspoon garlic powder

½ teaspoon ground cumin

2 cups shredded romaine lettuce

1 cup canned pinto beans, rinsed

1 ripe avocado, diced

¼ cup pico de gallo or fresh salsa

¼ cup shredded Cheddar or Monterey Jack cheese

Lime wedges for serving

instructions

Beat cauliflower in a food processor until cleaved into rice-size pieces. In a large skillet, heat 2 tablespoons of oil to medium-high heat. Salt to 1/4 teaspoon and add the cauliflower. Cook for about 5 minutes, stirring occasionally, until the cauliflower is soft. Keep warm by covering up.

In the upper third of the oven, place a rack; turn the broiler on high. Spray cooking spray all over a large baking sheet with a rim.

Season chicken with the leftover 1/4 teaspoon salt. Broil for nine minutes on the prepared baking sheet.

In the meantime, in a small bowl, combine the chipotles, garlic powder, cumin, and the remaining 1 tablespoon of oil.

Turn the chicken over, brush with the chipotle coating and keep cooking until a moment later the thermometer embedded in the thickest part enlists 165 degrees F, 8 to 10 minutes more. Cut into bite-sized pieces on a clean cutting board after transferring.

Fill each bowl with half a cup of cauliflower rice, half a cup of chicken, lettuce, and beans, one quarter of an avocado, and one tablespoon each of cheese and pico de gallo (or salsa) With a lime wedge, serve.

6. Sandwich with Chicken, Tomato, and Avocado
In this solid chicken sandwich recipe, the avocado is crushed to make a sound smooth spread.

Cook Time: 5 mins
Total Time: 5 mins
Servings: 1

Yield: 1 sandwich each

Ingredients

2 slices multigrain bread

¼ ripe avocado

3 ounces cooked boneless, skinless chicken breast, sliced (see Tip)

2 slices tomato

Instructions

Toast the bread Squash avocado with a fork and spread onto one piece of toast. Top with the second piece of toast, tomato, and chicken.

Tip: You can use poached chicken in a recipe if you don't have cooked chicken. In a skillet or saucepan, place chicken breasts without bones and skin. Cover with water that has been lightly salted and bring to a boil. Cover, diminish intensity to a stew and cook until presently not pink in the center, 10 to 15 minutes, contingent upon size. (Eight ounces crude boneless, skinless chicken bosom yields around 1 cup cut, diced or destroyed cooked chicken.)

7. The Best Sandwich With Rotisserie Chicken

A dressing based on muhammara, a Middle Eastern sauce made from breadcrumbs, walnuts, and spices, gives this rotisserie chicken sandwich its flavor. By including almonds in the mixture, we gave it our own unique spin. Additionally, cashews can be used for a creamier outcome. The sauce that is left over can be used as a dip for vegetables or bread, or as a condiment on just about anything.

Active Time: 10 mins

Total Time: 10 mins

Servings: 4

Ingredients

1 (12-ounce) jar marinated roasted red peppers, drained

⅔ cup unsalted roasted almonds or cashews

¼ cup panko breadcrumbs

2 tablespoons extra-virgin olive oil

1 tablespoon fresh lemon juice

1 ½ teaspoons balsamic vinegar

1 teaspoon honey

1 teaspoon salt

½ teaspoon ground cumin

½ teaspoon ground coriander

¼ teaspoon crushed red pepper

¼ cup mayonnaise

12 ounces shredded rotisserie chicken (about 3 cups)

1 cup loosely packed Little Gem lettuce leaves

8 slices whole-grain bread, toasted if desired

Instructions

In a little food processor, join the crushed red pepper, almonds (or cashews), panko, oil, lemon juice, vinegar, honey, salt, cumin, and coriander. Process until smooth and velvety in one to two minutes (it's okay if some irregularities remain). Place half of the mixture in a medium bowl; Mix in the mayonnaise by stirring. Save the leftover red pepper combination for another utilization.)

Chicken should be added to the dressing-filled bowl. Overlap in half to totally cover. Put lettuce leaves on four cuts of bread. Top with about 3/4 cup of the chicken mixture. On top, orchestrate the excess bread cuts. If desired, divide the sandwiches in half before serving.

Tip: For up to five days (Stage 1), separately refrigerate the muhammara and dressing in a hermetically sealed container.

8. 20-Minute Chicken Enchiladas

Speedy tip: Shred the chicken while the sauce is cooking. Add chopped jalapenos to the dish to add some heat.

Active Time: 20 mins

Total Time: 20 mins

Servings: 6

Ingredients

1 cup pre chopped onion

1 cup unsalted chicken stock (such as Swanson)

1 tablespoon all-purpose flour

1 ½ tablespoons chili powder

2 teaspoons ground cumin

¾ teaspoon garlic powder

½ teaspoon crushed red pepper

¼ teaspoon salt

1 (15-ounce) can unsalted tomato sauce

3 cups shredded skinless, boneless rotisserie chicken breast (about 15 ounces)

1 (15-ounce) can unsalted black beans, rinsed and drained

12 (6-inch) corn tortillas

Cooking spray

3 ounces pre shredded 4-cheese Mexican blend cheese (about 3/4 cup)

1 cup chopped tomato

¼ cup chopped fresh cilantro

6 tablespoons sour cream

Instructions

Stage 1:

Turn the broiler on high.

Step2:

In a medium saucepan, combine the onion, flour, chicken stock, chili powder, cumin, garlic powder, crushed red pepper, salt, and tomato sauce; Using a whisk, stir. Heat to the point of boiling over high intensity; cook for two minutes, or until the mixture becomes thick. Keep 1 1/2 cups of the sauce mixture. Add beans and chicken to the pan; cook for 2 minutes or until the chicken is completely warmed.

Step3:

Stack tortillas; Wrap the stack in damp paper towels and heat in the microwave for 25 seconds on HIGH. Place about a third of the chicken mixture in the middle of each tortilla; crease up. In a 13 x 9-inch glass or ceramic baking dish coated with cooking spray, arrange the tortillas seam-side down. Cover with the remaining sauce and cheese. Cook 3 minutes or until cheddar is delicately sautéed and sauce is effervescent. Garnish with cilantro and tomato. Present with acrid cream.

Dinner

1. Spaghetti with Quick Meat Sauce

Try this quick and easy spaghetti with meat sauce on a weeknight instead of opening a jar of sauce. Present with steamed broccoli and garlic bread. Eight servings can be obtained from the recipe. Cook 8 ounces of spaghetti and freeze the sauce if you only have four people for dinner.

Cook Time: 30 mins

Total Time: 30 mins

Servings: 8

Yield: 8 servings, 1 cup pasta & generous 3/4 cup sauce eac

Ingredients

1 pound whole-wheat spaghetti

2 teaspoons extra-virgin olive oil

1 large onion, finely chopped

1 large carrot, finely chopped

1 stalk celery, finely chopped

4 cloves garlic, minced

1 tablespoon Italian seasoning

1 pound lean ground beef

1 28-ounce can crushed tomatoes

¼ cup chopped flat-leaf parsley

½ teaspoon salt

½ cup grated Parmesan cheese

Instructions

Step 1:

Boil some water in a large pot. According to the package, cook the pasta for 8 to 10 minutes or until just tender. Drain.

Step 2:

In the meantime, heat oil in an enormous skillet over medium intensity. Cook the onion, carrot, and celery for 5 to 8 minutes, stirring occasionally, until the onion begins to brown.

Step 3:

Add the Italian seasoning and garlic; cook for about 30 seconds until fragrant. Cook beef for 3 to 5 minutes, breaking it up with a spoon and stirring, or until no longer pink. Increment intensity to high. Mix in tomatoes and cook until thickened, 4 to 6 minutes. Add salt and parsley and stir.

Step 4:

Serve the pasta with the sauce and cheese on top.

Tip for Preparing:

Refrigerate for up to three days or freeze for up to three months in an airtight container.

2. Steak with Glazed Carrots & Turnips

A pop of rosemary on the steak, a vigorous sear in a hot skillet, and a sweet-and-sour glaze on the vegetables make this cast-iron steak recipe perfect for elevating beef and vegetables to new heights. With some red wine and spinach that has been sautéed, serve.

Cook Time: 30 mins

Additional Time: 10 mins

Total Time: 40 mins

Servings: 4

Yield: 4 servings

Ingredients

2 tablespoons extra-virgin olive oil, divided

1 tablespoon butter

1 pound small carrots (about 5 inches long), halved lengthwise

1 pound turnips (about 3 medium), peeled and cut into thick matchsticks

¾ teaspoon salt, divided

¾ teaspoon ground pepper, divided

1 pound sirloin or top round steak, about 1 inch thick, trimmed

1 teaspoon minced fresh rosemary or 1/2 teaspoon dried

2 tablespoons brown sugar

1 tablespoon red-wine vinegar

Instructions

Stage 1:

Preheat the broiler to 450 degrees F.

Step 2:

In an enormous cast-iron skillet, heat 1 tablespoon of spread and oil over medium-high intensity. Salt and pepper the carrots and turnips with 1/4 teaspoon each and cook for 8 to 10 minutes, stirring occasionally, or until they begin to brown and become soft. On a plate, place.

Step 3:

After cutting the steak in half crosswise, rub rosemary and the remaining 1/2 teaspoon of salt and pepper on it. The skillet's excess 1 tablespoon of oil ought to be warmed to an extremely high temperature. Before adding the steak, cook it for about 2 minutes on each side. Move to an alternate plate.

Step 4:

Mix in the earthy-colored sugar after returning the vegetables to the skillet. Spread the vegetables over the steak. Warily move the compartment to the grill.

Step 5:

Broil for 8 to 10 minutes for medium-rare, or until the steak is cooked through and the vegetables are tender. Before cutting, transfer the steak to a clean cutting board and allow it to rest for five minutes. Sprinkle the vegetables with vinegar. Serve the steak with the vegetables.

3. Moroccan Skirt Steak with Roasted Pepper Couscous

When seared in a hot skillet, thin cuts of beef like skirt steak and sirloin steak cook quickly, making them ideal for busy weeknights. We love the amazing way the zesty Moroccan flavors on the steak supplement the sweet, cooked pepper-stuffed couscous. Prepare with: Salad with arugula and a bottle of Pinot Noir

Cook Time: 35 mins

Total Time: 35 mins

Servings: 4   Yield: 4 servings

Ingredients

2 medium bell peppers

1 teaspoon ground cumin

1 teaspoon ground coriander

¾ teaspoon salt

½ teaspoon ground turmeric

½ teaspoon ground cinnamon

½ teaspoon freshly ground pepper

1 whole lemon, plus more lemon wedges for garnish

1 teaspoon plus 1 tablespoon extra-virgin olive oil, divided

⅔ cup whole-wheat couscous

1 pound skirt steak (see Note) or sirloin steak, 3/4 to 1 inch thick, trimmed

2 tablespoons chopped green olives

Instructions

Step 1

Rack should be in the upper third of the oven; preheat the oven.

Step 2:

The bell peppers should be roasted for 10 to 15 minutes on a baking sheet under the broiler, turning once every 5 minutes, until they are charred and soft. Move to a dry cutting board; Cut the peppers into bite-sized pieces when they are cool enough to handle.

Step 3:

In the meantime, join cumin, coriander, salt, turmeric, cinnamon and pepper in a little bowl. Grate the lemon's zest into a fine powder. Juice the lemon into a 1-cup measure and add sufficient water to make 1 cup. Fill a little pan and add the lemon zing, 1 teaspoon of the flavor combination and 1 teaspoon olive oil. Heat to the point of boiling. Cover, add the couscous, stir, and let stand.

Step 4:

In a large skillet, preferably cast-iron, heat the remaining 1 tablespoon of oil until shimmering (but not smoking) over medium heat. Apply the remaining spice mixture to the steak on both sides. Cook the steak 2 to 3 minutes for each side and grill to perfection. Let lay on the cutting board for 5 minutes. Mix olives and the peppers into the couscous. Serve the steak with the couscous and, if desired, lemon wedges after it has been thinly sliced.

Note on the Ingredients: Skirt steak is a cut of beef that is thin, flavorful, and relatively inexpensive. Fajita steak is another name for it. Search for it in all around loaded general stores or request that your butcher request it for you.

Reduce Food Waste: A rimmed baking sheet is perfect for all that from broiling to getting unintentional dribbles and spills. Before each use, line your baking sheets with foil to make cleanup simple and to keep them in good shape.

4. Skillet Ravioli Lasagna

This simple back to front ravioli lasagna is a definitive weeknight solace food — no layering or blending bowls required. You are welcome to substitute ground turkey for the beef. Search for new mozzarella balls (additionally called "pearls") in the specialty cheddar segment of your supermarket.

Prep Time: 20 mins

Total Time: 20 mins

Servings: 6

Yield: 13 1/2 cups

Ingredients

1 (24 ounce) package frozen or refrigerated cheese ravioli

1 pound lean ground beef

1 ½ teaspoons dried oregano

½ teaspoon garlic powder

½ teaspoon salt

¼ teaspoon ground pepper

1 (28 ounce) can no-salt-added crushed tomatoes

¼ cup chopped fresh basil

8 ounces small fresh mozzarella balls, divided

Instructions

Stage 1 Preheat toaster. In a large pot, bring the water to a pustule. Cook the ravioli as directed on the package; channel and save

Stage 2 Over medium-high heat, deteriorate the ground beef with a rustic   ladle in a large cast- iron or toaster-safe skillet until it's cooked through, about 4 to 5 twinkles. Add swab, pepper, oregano, and garlic greasepaint to taste.

Stage 3:

Include basil and tomatoes; simmer for 5 minutes. Stir in half of the mozzarella balls and the cooked ravioli.

Stage 4:

Disperse the leftover mozzarella balls over the pasta. Cautiously move the container to the broiler. 2 to 3 minutes in the broiler will melt the cheese.

5. Strip Steaks with Smoky Cilantro Sauce and Simmered Vegetables

In this solid supper recipe, a cast-iron dish performs twofold responsibility via burning the steaks and broiling the vegetables. You don't like cilantro? Parsley would be a great addition to the sauce.

Cook Time: 40 mins

Additional Time: 10 mins

Total Time: 50 mins

Servings: 4

Yield: 4 servings

Ingredients

1 cup packed fresh cilantro

1 small fresh red chile, seeded and chopped

1 large clove garlic, finely grated

1 tablespoon tomato paste

2 teaspoons red-wine vinegar

1 teaspoon smoked paprika

½ teaspoon ground cumin

½ teaspoon brown sugar

5 tablespoons extra-virgin olive oil, divided

1 pound Brussels sprouts, trimmed and quartered

1 large sweet potato, peeled and cubed (1/2-inch)

¾ teaspoon salt, divided

½ teaspoon ground pepper, divided

2 8-ounce strip steaks, trimmed and halved

Instructions

Step 1

Preheat the roaster to 450 degreesF.

Step 2 In a small food processor, combine the cilantro, chili, garlic, tomato paste, ginger, paprika, cumin, brown sugar, and 2 soup spoons of oil painting. palpitation until smooth, scraping the sides as necessary. Place away.

Step 3 In a large cast- iron skillet, heat 2 soup spoons of the oil painting over medium-high heat. drop intensity to medium and add Brussels sprouts, yam and 1/4 tablespoon each swab and pepper. Cook, stirring constantly, for 9 to 12 twinkles or until nearly tender. Place on a plate.

Step 4 Steaks should be seasoned with the remaining 1/4 tablespoon pepper and 1/2 tablespoon swab. toast the redundant 1 teaspoon oil painting in the dish. Cook the steaks, one at a time, until browned, about one nanosecond.

Step 5   Settle the vegetables around the steaks in the dish. The steaks should be outgunned with half the redundant sauce. Move to the cookstove and dish until the steaks are wanted doneness, 8 to 10 twinkles for medium. Mix the leftover sauce into the vegetables and serve them with the steaks.

Tips for Preparing Get ready sauce(Stage 2) and chill for as long as 1 day.

6. Garlic-Lime Pork with Farro and Spinach

A zesty peanut butter-lime sauce pairs pork chops with farro and spinach in this straightforward main dish recipe. This meal can be prepared in just one skillet and takes less than 30 minutes to prepare.

Prep Time: 15 mins

Additional Time: 10 mins

Total Time: 25 mins

Servings: 4

Yield: 4 servings

Ingredients

3 tablespoons lime juice

1 tablespoon peanut butter or almond butter

4 cloves garlic, minced

1 ½ teaspoons honey

½ teaspoon salt

½ teaspoon black pepper

4 (8 ounce) bone-in pork chops, cut 3/4 to 1 inch thick and trimmed

4 teaspoons olive oil

1 8.5-ounce pouch cooked farro, such as Simply Balanced™

2 (5 ounce) packages fresh baby spinach

2 tablespoons chopped walnuts, toasted (see Tip) (Optional)

1 wedge Lime wedges

Instructions

Step 1:

Combine the peanut butter, honey, garlic, lime juice, 1/4 teaspoon each of salt and pepper in a small bowl. Sprinkle hacks with the leftover 1/4 teaspoon salt and pepper.

Step 2:

Heat 2 teaspoons of the oil in a 12-inch nonstick skillet on medium-high. Chops in; Cook, turning once, for 7 to 10 minutes or until a thermometer reads 145 degrees Fahrenheit. Eliminate from skillet; Keep warm by covering up.

Step 3:

Heat the remaining 2 teaspoons of oil in the same skillet to medium. Stir in the lime mixture to break up any crusty brown bits. Put farro in; cook and mix until grains are isolated. Add spinach; Cook and stir until spinach begins to wilt and is heated through. Sprinkle on additional pepper if desired.

Step 4:

With the farro mixture, serve the chops. Serve with lime wedges and sprinkle with walnuts if desired.

Tip:

Spread the nuts out in a shallow baking pan lined with parchment paper and heat the oven to 350 degrees Fahrenheit. Shaking the pan twice during baking, bake for 5 to 10 minutes or until golden.

7. Paprika Baked Pork Tenderloin with Potatoes and Broccoli

It's hard to believe that this sophisticated dish only requires one baking sheet to prepare. While the pork rests, whip together a simple red pepper sauce to finish this great and solid supper. The sauce would likewise be scrumptious with chicken. We're willing to wager that your kitchen playlist will feature a lot of this simple sheet-pan dinner recipe.

Prep Time: 25 mins

Additional Time: 20 mins

Total Time: 45 mins

Servings: 4

Yield: 4 servings

Ingredients

¾ pound Yukon Gold potatoes, scrubbed and cut into 1-inch pieces

1 medium red onion, cut into 1 inch pieces

2 tablespoons olive oil, divided

¾ teaspoon salt, divided

4 cups broccoli florets (about 1 lb.)

2 cloves garlic, peeled

1 ½ teaspoons smoked paprika

½ teaspoon ground pepper, divided

2 teaspoons Dijon mustard

1 (1 pound) pork tenderloin, trimmed

2 jarred roasted red bell peppers (6 oz.)

2 tablespoons low-fat sour cream or low-fat plain Greek yogurt

1 teaspoon lemon juice

Instructions

Step 1:

In the oven, place a large baking sheet with a rim; preheat to 425 degrees F.

Stage 2:

1 tablespoon each of onion and potatoes oil and 1/4 teaspoon salt in a medium bowl; throw to cover. Take the baking pan out of the oven; cover with cooking splash. On the pan, spread the potato mixture; cook for 15 minutes.

Step 3:

In the interim, consolidate broccoli, 2 tsp. olive oil, and 1/4 tsp. a medium bowl of salt; throw to cover. On a small piece of foil, arrange the garlic. Shower with the excess 1 tsp. oil; crease up into a little bundle. Combine 1/4 teaspoon paprika pepper, ground, and the remaining

1/4 teaspoon. in a small bowl, salt. Spread mustard all over pork. Cover with the paprika combination.

Step 4:

Eliminate the dish from the broiler. Move the potatoes and onions to one side and stir them. Place the pork close to the potatoes; On the other side of the pan, spread the broccoli. Place the garlic packet where there is room. In about 25 minutes, roast the pork until an instant-read thermometer inserted in the thickest part registers 145 degrees F.

Step 5:

Allow the pork to rest while you make the sauce: Transfer the garlic to a mini food processor or blender after carefully unwrapping it. Add cooked red peppers, harsh cream (or yogurt), lemon juice, and the excess 1/4 tsp. ground pepper. Blend till smooth.

Step 6:

Cut the pork into 12 cuts. Split the broccoli, potatoes, and pork among four plates. Shower the red pepper sauce over the top.

Review Page

To Florilegium,

I hope this message finds you in good health. I would like to respectfully ask for your opinion on my most recent book, "Losing weight for women: Achieving Your Ideal Weight with Simple Home Workouts." Your research and insights are really valuable to me, and I would be very grateful if you could dedicate a significant amount of time to reviewing what I have written. Your comments will help me to keep improving my work, regardless of whether you found the book enjoyable or possess constructive perception.

By giving your honest assessment, other albums will be better able to decide whether or not this book suits their needs and interests. Nevertheless, I would much appreciate it if you could take a moment to write a review on the website.

Your help is greatly appreciated.

Jasmin W. Alcantara

www.ingramcontent.com/pod-product-compliance
Lightning Source LLC
Chambersburg PA
CBHW070928260726
48661CB00003B/883